ANCIENT REMEDIES REVIVED

PLANT REMEDIES, MEDICINAL HERBS RECIPES, AND NATURAL HEALING KNOWLEDGE FROM NATIVE AMERICAN HERBALISM AND CHINESE TRADITIONAL MEDICINE

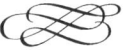

LEAF INSIGHT BOOKS

CONTENTS

Introduction	7
CHAPTER 1: FOUNDATIONS OF ANCIENT REMEDIES	11
The Historical Roots of Native American Medicine	12
The Foundations of Traditional Chinese Medicine	14
Comparing Native American and Traditional Chinese Medicinal Practices	17
The Role of Herbalism in Ancient Cultures	19
Essential Tools and Ingredients for Herbal Preparations	22
Understanding the Science Behind Herbal Remedies	25
CHAPTER 2: NATIVE AMERICAN REMEDIES AND RECIPES	29
Sacred Herbs of Native American Medicine	29
Preparing Herbal Teas for Common Ailments	31
Crafting Salves and Ointments from Native Plants	34
Traditional Remedies for Respiratory Health	36
The Use of Plants in Native American Rituals	38
Herbal Infusions for Digestive Wellness	40
CHAPTER 3: TRADITIONAL CHINESE MEDICINE REMEDIES	45
Key Herbs in Traditional Chinese Medicine	45
Preparing Decoctions for Immune Support	48
Herbal Remedies for Stress and Anxiety	50
Crafting Tinctures for Longevity and Vitality	53
The Role of Adaptogens in Chinese Medicine	55
Using Chinese Herbs in Daily Diets	58
CHAPTER 4: GLOBAL ANCIENT REMEDIES	61
Ayurvedic Herbs and Their Healing Properties	61
Ancient Egyptian Herbal Practices	64
Traditional African Plant Remedies	66
Indigenous Australian Bush Medicine	69

South American Herbal Healing Traditions ... 71
Ancient European Herbal Lore ... 73

CHAPTER 5: PRACTICAL APPLICATIONS OF HERBS ... 77
Herbal Baths and Their Benefits ... 77
Making Herbal Syrups for Cough and Cold ... 80
Crafting Essential Oils at Home ... 82
Homemade Herbal Lotions and Creams ... 85
Capsules and Tablets: Modern Takes on Ancient Remedies ... 88
Preparing Herbal Rubs for Pain Relief ... 90

CHAPTER 6: PREVENTATIVE HEALTH AND IMMUNITY ... 93
Daily Tonics for Immune Support ... 93
Seasonal Herbs for Cold and Flu Prevention ... 96
Herbal Remedies for Boosting Energy ... 99
Natural Detoxification with Herbs ... 101
Adaptogenic Herbs for Stress Management ... 103
Herbal Strategies for Anti-Aging ... 105

CHAPTER 7: SAFETY AND SUSTAINABILITY IN HERBAL MEDICINE ... 109
Identifying and Sourcing Quality Herbs ... 109
Safety Precautions and Potential Side Effects ... 113
Ethical Harvesting and Sustainable Practices ... 115
Integrating Modern Science with Traditional Wisdom ... 117
Creating a Sustainable Herbal Garden ... 120
Navigating Herbal Interactions with Conventional Medications ... 123

CHAPTER 8: BUILDING A HOLISTIC LIFESTYLE ... 127
Daily Rituals for Holistic Health ... 127
Combining Herbal Remedies with Meditation and Yoga ... 130
Dietary Changes to Complement Herbal Treatments ... 132
Mind-Body Connection and Herbal Medicine ... 134
Building a Community Around Herbal Practices ... 136
Continuing Your Journey: Further Resources and Reading ... 138

Conclusion 141
References 145

© **Copyright 2024** - **All rights reserved.** The content contained within this book may not be reproduced, duplicated, or transmitted without direct written permission from the author or the publisher. Under no circumstances will any blame or legal responsibility be held against the publisher or author for any damages, reparation, or monetary loss due to the information contained within this book, either directly or indirectly.

Legal Notice: This book is copyright-protected. It is only for personal use. You cannot amend, distribute, sell, use, quote, or paraphrase any part of the content within this book without the consent of the author or publisher.

Disclaimer Notice: Please note the information contained within this document is for educational and entertainment purposes only. All efforts have been executed to present accurate, up-to-date, reliable, and complete information. No warranties of any kind are declared or implied. Readers acknowledge that the author is not engaged in the rendering of legal, financial, medical, or professional advice. The content within this book has been derived from various sources. Please consult a licensed professional before attempting any techniques outlined in this book.

By reading this document, the reader agrees that under no circumstances is the author responsible for any direct or indirect losses incurred as a result of the use of the information contained within this document, including, but not limited to, errors, omissions, or inaccuracies.

INTRODUCTION

Years ago, I found myself standing in a small, dimly lit apothecary in the heart of an ancient village. The shelves were lined with jars of dried herbs, roots, and colorful powders. The air was thick with the scent of earth and mystery. An elderly woman, her hands weathered but gentle, handed me a cup of tea brewed from plants I'd never heard of. With my first sip, I felt a warmth and a sense of calm wash over me. That moment ignited a passion for the ancient remedies and the wisdom they carried.

This book is born from that spark. Its purpose is to revive ancient healing practices from Native American and Traditional Chinese Medicine, along with remedies from other ancient civilizations. The aim is to provide you with a guide that bridges the old and the new, offering practical applications for these time-honored traditions in our modern world.

Herbal medicine has a rich history that stretches back thousands of years. Native American tribes relied on the healing power of plants to treat ailments and maintain health. Traditional Chinese Medicine has been practiced for millennia with its intricate understanding of the body's energy systems. Ancient Egypt, India, and other civilizations also developed their own herbal traditions. These practices were passed down through generations, often through oral tradition, and have stood the test of time.

Today, we are witnessing a resurgence of interest in natural and holistic health solutions. Modern health challenges and a growing desire for sustainable living have led many to seek alternatives to conventional medicine. Ancient remedies offer a path to wellness grounded in tradition and supported by modern science.

This book is structured into three main sections. The first section focuses on Native American remedies. You'll discover the historical context, specific herbs, and preparation methods used by various tribes. The second section delves into Traditional Chinese Medicine, exploring its complex system of diagnosis and treatment. The third section offers remedies from other ancient cultures, including Egypt, India, and more. Each section provides historical insights and practical applications for integrating these remedies into your daily life.

Exploring these ancient remedies can help you better understand natural healing methods. This knowledge empowers you to take charge of your health and well-being. The recipes and techniques you'll find here are designed to be easy to follow, making it simple for you to incorporate them into your routine.

Leaf Insight Books has dedicated many years of research to helping people achieve a holistic, healthy lifestyle. Our passion for herbal medicine is rooted in a desire to provide reputable, easy-to-follow guidance that anyone can benefit from. We have spent years researching and practicing these ancient remedies, and I am thrilled to share that knowledge with you.

In this book, you will find a blend of historical insights, practical recipes, and modern scientific validations of ancient practices. You can trust that the content is backed by thorough research and a deep respect for the traditions it represents. My goal is to offer you a resource that is both informative and transformative.

As you turn these pages, I invite you to embark on a journey of self-discovery and healing. Embrace the wisdom of ancient remedies and experience the transformative power of natural health solutions. Whether you are seeking relief from a specific ailment or looking to enhance your overall well-being, these time-tested practices offer valuable tools for your journey.

Let us step together into the world of ancient remedies, where the old meets the new, and the wisdom of the past enriches the present. Welcome to a journey of natural healing and holistic wellness.

CHAPTER 1: FOUNDATIONS OF ANCIENT REMEDIES

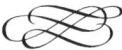

When I was a child, my grandmother would tell me stories of the "plant doctors" who lived in our village long before modern medicine. She spoke of how they could heal with just the touch of a leaf, the whisper of a chant, and the brewing of a simple tea. I remember the way her eyes would light up, filled with respect and awe for these ancient healers. This fascination with plant-based healing took root in me, leading to a lifelong passion for understanding and reviving these ancient remedies.

In this chapter, we will dive into the rich history and cultural significance of Native American medicine. We'll explore the foundational practices that have been passed down through generations, focusing on the oral traditions, shamanic beliefs, and community roles that shaped these healing methods. Additionally, we'll examine the historical periods that influenced Native American medicinal practices and highlight the key plants that were central to their healing traditions.

THE HISTORICAL ROOTS OF NATIVE AMERICAN MEDICINE

Native American medicine is deeply rooted in oral traditions that have preserved its knowledge for centuries. Elders and healers passed down their wisdom through stories, songs, and rituals, ensuring that each generation retained the knowledge of their ancestors. This oral tradition was not just about transferring information; it was a way to maintain a spiritual connection to the land and the plants that provided healing.

Shamanism played a crucial role in Native American medicine. Shamans, often regarded as spiritual leaders, entered trance states to communicate with the spirit world, seeking guidance and healing for their communities. They believed that illness was often a result of spiritual imbalance or malevolent forces, and healing required addressing these spiritual aspects. Through ceremonies, chants, and rituals, shamans restored harmony and balance within the individual and the community.

Community healers, often referred to as medicine men or women, were highly respected figures within their tribes. They possessed extensive knowledge of herbal remedies, spiritual practices, and physical healing techniques. These healers treated various ailments, from common colds to more severe conditions. They would often use a combination of herbal medicine, spiritual rituals, and hands-on healing to address the needs of their community.

Sacred rituals and ceremonies were integral to Native American healing practices. These ceremonies often involved the use of specific plants, chants, and dances to invoke healing energies. For example, the sweat lodge ceremony, a purification ritual, utilized steam and medicinal herbs to cleanse the body and spirit. Similarly, the use of smudging with sage and sweetgrass was believed to purify the space and ward off negative energies.

The history of Native American medicine can be divided into several key periods. In the pre-Columbian era, indigenous knowledge thrived, with tribes using a vast array of plants for medicinal purposes. This period saw the development of complex herbal systems and a deep understanding of the healing properties of various plants.

The arrival of European colonizers brought significant changes to Native American healing practices. Colonization led to the suppression of traditional knowledge and the introduction of new diseases. However, despite these challenges, Native American communities continued to preserve their medicinal traditions. Many tribes adapted by integrating some of the new plants and practices introduced by Europeans while maintaining the core elements of their traditional healing methods.

In modern times, there has been a resurgence of interest in Native American medicine. Efforts to preserve and revive these ancient practices have gained momentum, with many Native American communities actively working to document and pass down their traditional knowledge. This revival is not only about preserving cultural heritage but also about offering sustainable and holistic health solutions for future generations.

Several plants hold a significant place in Native American medicine. Sage, sweetgrass, and cedar are considered sacred herbs used for purification and protection. Echinacea, known for its immune-boosting properties, was widely used to treat infections. Willow bark, often referred to as "nature's aspirin," was used for its pain-relieving properties. These plants, among many others, formed the cornerstone of Native American herbal medicine.

The geography and climate of different tribal territories influenced regional variations in medicinal practices. Tribes in the Plains, Southwest, and Eastern Woodlands each had unique healing traditions based on the plants available in their regions. For instance, tribes in the Plains region used plants like yarrow and prairie sage, while those in the Southwest relied on desert plants such as yucca and mesquite. In the Eastern Woodlands, tribes utilized a variety of forest plants, including ginseng and goldenseal.

Understanding these regional differences is crucial for appreciating the diversity and richness of Native American medicine. Each tribe's knowledge and practices reflect its deep connection to the land and its ability to adapt to its specific environment. This regional approach to healing underscores the importance of sustainable and locally sourced herbal remedies.

The historical roots of Native American medicine offer a profound understanding of how ancient cultures viewed health and healing. Through oral traditions, shamanic practices, community healers, and sacred ceremonies, Native American tribes developed a holistic approach to medicine that addressed the physical, spiritual, and emotional aspects of health. By exploring these traditions, we can gain valuable insights into the timeless wisdom of natural healing and apply these practices to our lives today.

THE FOUNDATIONS OF TRADITIONAL CHINESE MEDICINE

Traditional Chinese Medicine (TCM) is deeply rooted in the philosophical concepts of Yin and Yang, the Five Elements, and the vital energy known as Qi. These principles form the foundation of TCM, guiding its diagnostic and treatment practices. The concept of Yin and Yang represents the duality present in all things. Yin embodies qualities such as darkness, cold, and passivity, while Yang represents light, warmth, and activity. Health is achieved by maintaining a dynamic balance between these two forces. An imbalance leads to illness, and TCM aims to restore harmony by adjusting the levels of Yin and Yang within the body.

The Five Elements Theory further enriches TCM's approach by categorizing all natural phenomena into five groups: wood, fire, earth, metal, and water. Each element corresponds to specific organs, emotions, and seasons. For example, the liver is associated with wood, the heart with fire, and so on. This theory helps practitioners understand the complex interrelationships within the body and their impact on health. It explains how different elements promote or control each other, thereby maintaining a balanced system. This holistic view allows for targeted treatments that address the root causes of ailments rather than just the symptoms.

Central to TCM is the concept of Qi, the vital energy that flows through the body. Qi is considered the life force that powers both physical and mental activities. It circulates through channels known as meridians, nourishing organs and tissues. Proper flow and balance of Qi are crucial for maintaining health. When Qi is deficient or blocked, it leads to disease. TCM treatments aim to regulate and harmonize the flow of Qi, ensuring that it moves freely and efficiently. Techniques like acupuncture, herbal medicine, and Qi Gong exercises are employed to balance Qi and restore health.

The historical development of TCM is marked by significant milestones, beginning with ancient texts like the Huangdi Neijing or the Yellow Emperor's Inner Canon. This foundational text, dating back to the Warring States period (475-221 BCE), laid the groundwork for TCM theories and practices. It covers various aspects of medicine, including anatomy, physiology, diagnosis, and treatment. The Huangdi Neijing remains a cornerstone of TCM, and its teachings are still relevant today. Over the centuries, other influential figures like Zhang Zhongjing and Sun Simiao contributed to the evolution of TCM. Zhang Zhongjing, often called the "Hippocrates of China," authored the Shang Han Lun (Treatise on Cold Damage), a seminal work on febrile diseases. Sun Simiao, known as the "King of Medicine," compiled the Qian Jin Yao Fang (Essential Prescriptions Worth a Thousand Gold), a comprehensive medical encyclopedia.

The Tang (618-907 CE) and Song (960-1279 CE) Dynasties were pivotal in codifying TCM practices. During these periods, medical texts were systematically compiled, and medical schools were established, ensuring the dissemination and standardization of TCM knowledge.

The Tang Dynasty saw the creation of the first official pharmacopeia, while the Song Dynasty further refined diagnostic techniques and herbal prescriptions. These advancements cemented TCM's place in Chinese culture and its enduring legacy.

Several medicinal herbs hold a prominent place in TCM. Ginseng (Ren Shen) is renowned for its ability to boost vitality and energy. It is often used to combat fatigue and enhance overall well-being. Astragalus (Huang Qi) is another vital herb known for its immune-boosting properties. It strengthens the body's defenses and is commonly used in preventive medicine. Licorice Root (Gan Cao) serves as a harmonizer in herbal formulas, enhancing the effects of other herbs and reducing potential side effects. These herbs, among many others, form the backbone of TCM's herbal pharmacopeia.

TCM employs various diagnostic and treatment techniques to address health issues. Pulse diagnosis is a critical diagnostic tool involving the examination of the radial pulse at three positions on

CHAPTER 1: FOUNDATIONS OF ANCIENT REMEDIES

each wrist. Each position corresponds to different organs, and variations in pulse quality provide insights into the patient's condition. This method allows practitioners to identify imbalances and tailor treatments accordingly. Acupuncture and moxibustion are key treatment modalities in TCM. Acupuncture involves inserting fine needles into specific points along the meridians to regulate Qi flow and alleviate pain. Moxibustion, the burning of moxa (dried mugwort) near the skin, warms and stimulates these points, enhancing the therapeutic effects of acupuncture.

Herbal prescriptions are meticulously formulated to address individual needs. Practitioners select herbs based on their properties and the patient's specific condition, combining them to create a balanced and effective remedy. These prescriptions are tailored to restore harmony within the body, addressing the root causes of illness.

COMPARING NATIVE AMERICAN AND TRADITIONAL CHINESE MEDICINAL PRACTICES

Native American and Traditional Chinese Medicine (TCM) both embrace holistic health approaches, viewing the body as an interconnected system where physical, emotional, and spiritual elements work in harmony. This shared philosophy underscores that true health comes from balance and integration. However, their conceptualizations of vital energy differ. Native American traditions often speak of "Spirit," a life force that connects individuals to the Earth and the cosmos. In contrast, TCM introduces the concept of Qi, a dynamic energy that flows through the body's meridians, crucial for maintaining health. While both traditions emphasize balance and harmony, TCM's Yin-Yang theory and Five Elements framework add layers of complexity to this understanding, explaining how seemingly opposite forces and elemental interactions govern bodily functions and overall well-being.

When it comes to the use of medicinal plants, each tradition has developed a rich pharmacopeia tailored to its unique environment and cultural context. In Native American medicine, plants like sage, sweetgrass, and cedar hold profound ceremonial significance and are used for purification and protection. The methods of preparation often involve smudging or creating infusions that are imbued with spiritual intent. TCM, on the other hand, employs herbs such as ginseng (Ren Shen) for boosting vitality, astragalus (Huang Qi) for immune support, and licorice root (Gan Cao) to harmonize herbal formulas. These herbs are typically prepared as decoctions, teas, and tinctures, guided by precise principles to balance Qi and restore health. The cultural significance of these plants is also paramount, with many TCM herbs linked to ancient legends and traditional beliefs, much like their Native American counterparts.

Diagnostic methods in both traditions reflect their unique philosophies. Native American healers often rely on spiritual and shamanic guidance to diagnose ailments. They might enter trance states, perform rituals, or interpret dreams to understand the root causes of illness. This approach combines physical observation with a deep connection to the spiritual realm. In contrast, TCM employs detailed physical examinations, including tongue and pulse diagnosis, to assess the body's internal state. Pulse diagnosis in TCM involves feeling the pulse at three positions on each wrist, each position corresponding to different organs and bodily functions. The quality, strength, and rhythm of the pulse provide insights into the patient's health, allowing for a comprehensive understanding and targeted treatment plan.

Treatment approaches in Native American and TCM traditions also show fascinating similarities and differences. Both systems use herbal remedies, but their formulations and applications vary. Native American healers might create a poultice from willow bark to relieve pain, combining the plant's natural properties with spiritual rituals to enhance its effectiveness. TCM practitioners formulate complex herbal prescriptions tailored to the individual's unique condition, balancing various herbs to achieve harmony within the body. Non-herbal treatments further distinguish these traditions. Acupuncture, a cornerstone of TCM, involves inserting fine needles into specific points to regulate Qi flow and alleviate ailments. Moxibustion, which uses the heat from burning moxa to stimulate acupuncture points, complements this practice. Native American healing, meanwhile, incorporates spiritual ceremonies such as the sweat lodge, where steam and medicinal herbs are used to cleanse and heal both body and spirit.

Both traditions integrate the body, mind, and spirit in their healing practices, recognizing that true wellness extends beyond the physical. This holistic approach resonates deeply in today's world, where many seek alternatives to purely biomedical treatments. By understanding and appreciating these ancient practices, we can enrich our modern health practices, finding balance and harmony in a complex, fast-paced world.

THE ROLE OF HERBALISM IN ANCIENT CULTURES

Herbalism has been a cornerstone of daily life and health practices in ancient cultures, deeply woven into the fabric of their existence. Herbalists and healers were often revered members of their communities, entrusted with the knowledge and skills to treat ailments and promote well-being. These individuals were more than just medical practitioners; they were keepers of ancestral wisdom, passing down their expertise through generations. In many cultures, the role of the herbalist was hereditary, with knowledge transferred from parent to child through hands-on training and storytelling. This ensured the continuity of valuable healing traditions and maintained the health of the community.

Cultural rituals and ceremonies involving herbs were integral to the social and spiritual life of ancient peoples. In many societies, herbs were not merely medicinal but also sacred, used in rituals to honor deities, mark significant life events, or seek divine intervention for health and prosperity. For example, ancient Egyptians used herbs like frankincense and myrrh in religious ceremonies and embalming practices, believing that these plants had both earthly and spiritual benefits. Similarly, in ancient India, Ayurvedic rituals often included the use of herbs like tulsi and neem to purify the body and mind, aligning the individual with cosmic energies.

The transmission of herbal knowledge was a vital aspect of preserving these traditions. Oral traditions played a significant role, with elders sharing their wisdom through stories, chants, and practical demonstrations. Written texts also became crucial in documenting herbal practices. For instance, the Ebers Papyrus, an ancient Egyptian medical text dating back to around 1550 BCE, contains extensive information on herbal remedies and their uses. This text is one of the earliest records of medical knowledge, showing the sophisticated understanding of plant-based medicine in ancient Egypt.

Ancient India contributed immensely to herbal medicine through Ayurveda, a system that emphasizes balance and harmony in the body. Ayurvedic texts like the Charaka Samhita and Sushruta Samhita, written over two thousand years ago, offer detailed descriptions of various herbs, their properties, and their

CHAPTER 1: FOUNDATIONS OF ANCIENT REMEDIES 21

applications. These texts provided a comprehensive guide to health and healing, influencing not only Indian medicine but also other medical traditions around the world.

In ancient Greece and Rome, herbalism was a well-developed field, with practitioners like Hippocrates and Galen documenting the medicinal properties of numerous plants. The Greek physician Dioscorides compiled "De Materia Medica," a five-volume work that became a cornerstone of herbal medicine in Europe for centuries. This text detailed the identification, preparation, and therapeutic uses of over 600 plants, showcasing the extensive botanical knowledge of the time.

The preservation and transmission of herbal knowledge have been influenced significantly by trade routes. The Silk Road, for example, facilitated the exchange of medicinal plants and herbal knowledge between East and West. Traders and travelers brought new plants and healing practices to different regions, enriching local traditions with foreign influences. This exchange of knowledge helped to create a more interconnected and diverse understanding of herbal medicine.

In modern times, there has been a renewed interest in documenting and preserving ancient herbal knowledge. Efforts to revive traditional practices are seen in various parts of the world, with scholars and practitioners working to compile and translate ancient texts, conduct scientific research, and promote sustainable herbal practices. This revival is not just about preserving history but also about finding effective and natural solutions for contemporary health challenges.

Geography has always played a crucial role in shaping herbal practices. The availability of plant species in different regions determined the types of herbs used and their applications. In tropical climates, for example, plants with cooling properties were often utilized to counteract the heat, while in colder regions, warming herbs were preferred. This adaptation to local climates and ecosystems highlights the ingenuity and resourcefulness of ancient herbalists.

Ancient Egyptians had access to a diverse range of plants in the fertile Nile Valley, which they used extensively in their medicinal practices. Herbs like aloe vera, castor oil, and garlic were staples in their medical toolkit. In contrast, the arid landscapes of ancient Mesopotamia required the use of hardy, drought-resistant plants like licorice and juniper. These regional differences in plant availability and environmental conditions led to the development of unique herbal traditions, each tailored to the specific needs and resources of their respective cultures.

Herbalism in ancient cultures was not just about treating illnesses; it was a holistic approach to health that integrated the physical, spiritual, and environmental aspects of well-being. This multifaceted approach ensured that herbal practices were sustainable, culturally relevant, and deeply connected to the natural world. By understanding the role of herbalism in these ancient cultures, we can appreciate the depth and richness of their knowledge and apply these timeless principles to our own lives.

ESSENTIAL TOOLS AND INGREDIENTS FOR HERBAL PREPARATIONS

In the world of herbal medicine, the tools you use can significantly impact the effectiveness of your remedies. One of the most iconic tools is the mortar and pestle. This ancient device, consisting of a bowl (mortar) and a grinding tool (pestle), is essential for crushing and grinding herbs. The manual grinding process helps release the plant's active compounds, making them more accessible for your preparations. Whether you're making a simple herbal tea or a complex salve, the mortar and pestle will be your reliable companion in ensuring that your herbs are finely ground and ready for use.

Strainers and cheesecloth are indispensable when it comes to preparing tinctures and infusions. These tools allow you to separate the liquid extract from the plant material, ensuring a smooth and clear final product. Strainers come in various sizes and mesh types, making them versatile for different herbal preparations. Cheesecloth, a loosely woven cotton fabric, is particularly useful for straining thicker infusions and decoctions. It can also be used to create herbal bundles for baths or compresses. These tools ensure that your herbal remedies are pure and free from unwanted plant particles.

Glass jars and bottles are crucial for storing your herbal preparations. Glass is a non-reactive material, meaning it won't interact with the herbal compounds and alter their properties. Amber or cobalt blue glass jars are particularly beneficial as they protect your preparations from light, which can degrade the potency of the herbs. These containers are perfect for storing tinctures, oils, and dried herbs. Proper storage is key to maintaining the efficacy of your remedies. Investing in quality glass jars and bottles will ensure that your herbal creations remain potent and effective.

When it comes to the basic ingredients used in herbal remedies, base oils, and alcohol play a foundational role. Base oils, such as olive oil, coconut oil, and almond oil, serve as carriers for the medicinal properties of herbs. They are used in making infusions, salves, and ointments. These oils not only extract the active compounds from the herbs but also provide moisturizing and nourishing benefits for the skin. Alcohol, typically vodka or brandy, is used in making tinctures. It acts as a solvent that extracts and preserves the medicinal constituents of the herbs, resulting in a concentrated liquid form that is easy to use and has a long shelf life.

Beeswax is another fundamental ingredient, especially in the making of salves and balms. This natural wax, produced by honeybees, adds a thick and stable consistency to your preparations. It also provides protective and soothing properties, making it ideal for skin applications. Beeswax helps to seal in moisture and create a barrier against environmental irritants. It also enhances the shelf life of your salves and balms by preventing the growth of bacteria and mold. The subtle honey scent that beeswax imparts to your creations is an added bonus, making your remedies pleasant to use.

Common herbs like chamomile, lavender, and peppermint are staples in many herbal preparations due to their versatility and wide range of benefits. Chamomile is known for its calming and anti-inflammatory properties, making it useful in teas, infusions, and skin treatments. Lavender offers soothing and antiseptic benefits, perfect for relaxation blends and topical applications. With its invigorating and cooling effects, peppermint is excellent in digestive aids and respiratory remedies. These herbs, among others, form the backbone of many herbal preparations, providing a foundation for creating effective and holistic remedies.

The methods of preparation in herbal medicine are diverse, each tailored to extract the maximum benefit from the herbs. Infusion and decoction techniques are commonly used for making teas and medicinal beverages. Infusions involve steeping delicate plant parts like leaves and flowers in hot water, while decoctions require simmering tougher plant materials like roots and bark to extract their medicinal properties. These methods are simple yet effective, allowing you to harness the healing power of herbs in a drinkable form.

Making tinctures and extracts involves soaking herbs in a solvent like alcohol or vinegar to create a concentrated liquid remedy. This method preserves the active compounds of the herbs, resulting in a potent extract that can be used in small doses. Tinctures are highly versatile and can be added to teas, taken directly, or used in various recipes. Crafting salves, balms, and ointments involves infusing herbs into oils and then combining them with beeswax or other thickening agents. These preparations are used for topical applications, providing a protective and healing barrier on the skin.

Quality and sourcing are paramount in herbal medicine. Selecting organic and sustainably sourced herbs ensures that your remedies are free from harmful pesticides and chemicals. It also supports ethical farming practices that protect the environment. Verifying the credibility of suppliers is equally important. Look for suppliers who provide transparency about their sourcing practices and offer quality certifications. Proper storage techniques, for example, keeping herbs in airtight containers away from light and moisture, help maintain their potency. By prioritizing quality and ethical sourcing, you ensure that your herbal preparations are both effective and environmentally responsible.

UNDERSTANDING THE SCIENCE BEHIND HERBAL REMEDIES

Scientific principles underpin the efficacy of herbal medicine, bridging ancient wisdom with modern understanding. At the heart of this science is phytochemistry, the study of the active compounds in plants. These compounds, such as alkaloids, flavonoids, and terpenes, are the chemical powerhouses that give herbs their medicinal properties. For instance, alkaloids like morphine from the poppy plant have potent pain-relieving effects, while flavonoids found in chamomile provide anti-inflammatory benefits. These active compounds interact with our body's systems in complex ways, influencing physiological processes and promoting healing.

Herbs interact with the body's systems through a variety of mechanisms. For example, some herbs modulate the immune system, either boosting its activity or calming it down in cases of autoimmune disorders. Echinacea, a well-known immune stimulant, enhances the activity of white blood cells, helping the body fend off infections. Other herbs, like valerian, affect the nervous system by interacting with neurotransmitter receptors to promote relaxation and improve sleep. Understanding these interactions helps us appreciate how herbs can support the body's natural healing processes.

Secondary metabolites, the byproducts of plant metabolism, play a crucial role in herbal medicine. These compounds, which include essential oils and resins, often serve as the plant's defense mechanisms against pests and diseases. When used in herbal remedies, secondary metabolites provide therapeutic benefits, such as antimicrobial and antioxidant effects. For instance, the essential oil of tea trees has potent antibacterial properties, making it an effective remedy for skin infections. These metabolites demonstrate the intricate ways in which plants have evolved to protect themselves and, in turn, offer healing benefits to humans.

Modern scientific research has increasingly validated the traditional uses of herbs. Clinical trials have shown the efficacy of specific herbs in treating various conditions. For example, studies on St. John's Wort have demonstrated its effectiveness in alleviating mild to moderate depression, comparable to conventional antidepressants but with fewer side effects. Similarly, ginkgo biloba has been shown to improve cognitive function in individuals with dementia. These studies provide empirical support for the traditional uses of these herbs, bridging the gap between ancient practices and modern medicine.

Research also explores the safety and potential side effects of herbal remedies. While many herbs are generally safe, some can cause adverse reactions, especially when used improperly. For instance, excessive consumption of licorice root can lead to elevated blood pressure and potassium imbalances. By understanding these risks, we can use herbs more safely and effectively. Modern research often focuses on identifying safe dosage ranges and potential interactions with conventional medications, providing valuable guidelines for integrating herbal remedies into contemporary healthcare.

Integration of traditional knowledge with modern science enhances the credibility and effectiveness of herbal medicine. Scientists collaborate with traditional healers to document and study indigenous practices, preserving this knowledge for future generations. This collaboration ensures that traditional wisdom is respected and validated through scientific rigor. For example, the traditional use of turmeric in Ayurveda for its anti-inflammatory properties has been confirmed by numerous studies, highlighting curcumin, its active compound, as a potent anti-inflammatory agent. This integration enriches our understanding and application of herbal remedies in a modern context.

Addressing common misconceptions about herbal medicine is essential for informed use. One prevalent myth is that natural always means safe. While herbs are natural, they are not free from risks. Some can interact with medications or cause allergic reactions. Understanding these risks and using herbs responsibly is crucial. Another misconception is about dosage and potency. Just because an herb is natural doesn't mean it can be consumed in unlimited quantities. Proper dosing is essential to avoid toxicity and ensure effectiveness. Additionally, the idea that herbs are cure-alls is misleading. While herbs can support health and alleviate symptoms, they are not panaceas. They work best as part of a holistic approach to health, complementing other treatments and lifestyle changes.

Integrating herbal remedies with conventional medicine requires careful consideration. Consult healthcare professionals before starting any herbal regimen to ensure it is safe and appropriate for your specific condition. This is especially important if you are taking prescription medications, as some herbs can interact with drugs, either enhancing or diminishing their effects. For example, St. John's Wort can reduce the effectiveness of birth control pills and certain antidepressants. Monitoring and adjusting dosages under professional guidance can help avoid adverse interactions and optimize the benefits of both herbal and conventional treatments.

In conclusion, understanding the science behind herbal remedies enhances our ability to use them safely and effectively. By appreciating the biological and chemical mechanisms of herbs, validating traditional uses through modern research, and addressing common misconceptions, we can integrate these ancient practices into our contemporary healthcare routines. This holistic approach empowers us to take charge of our health, blending the wisdom of the past with the advancements of the present.

CHAPTER 2: NATIVE AMERICAN REMEDIES AND RECIPES

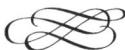

The first time I encountered the profound healing power of Native American herbs, I was on a hiking trip through the majestic Rockies. I had developed a stubborn cough, and a local guide handed me a small bundle of sage, instructing me to breathe in its smoke. Almost instantly, the soothing warmth and earthy aroma began to ease my discomfort. That simple act sparked a lifelong fascination with the sacred herbs of Native American medicine, leading me to explore their deep cultural significance and remarkable healing properties.

SACRED HERBS OF NATIVE AMERICAN MEDICINE

In Native American culture, sacred herbs play an essential role in both spirituality and healing. These plants are not merely seen as physical remedies but as spiritual allies that connect individuals to the divine and the natural world. Sage, for example, is widely revered for its purification and protection rituals. When burnt, its smoke is believed to cleanse spaces of negative energy and create a protective barrier. This ritual, known as smudging, is used in various ceremonies and personal practices to promote spiritual and emotional well-being.

Sweetgrass, another sacred herb, symbolizes positivity and kindness. Often referred to as the "hair of Mother Earth," sweetgrass is braided and used in healing rituals to attract good spirits and positive energy. The sweet, vanilla-like scent of the burning braid is said to invite peace and harmony into the environment, making it a staple in many traditional ceremonies. Tobacco, held in high esteem, is used in offerings and prayers. It is considered a sacred plant that facilitates communication with the spirit world. In many Native American traditions, tobacco is offered to the spirits as a sign of respect and gratitude. Cedar, known as "the grandfather medicine," is used for its cleansing and medicinal properties. Burning cedar during prayers and ceremonies is believed to purify the air and protect against illness. Its leaves and bark are also used in various medicinal preparations to treat colds, fevers, and rheumatic symptoms.

The medicinal properties of these sacred herbs are as diverse as their spiritual uses. Cedar, for instance, possesses powerful anti-inflammatory properties, making it effective in treating joint pain and respiratory ailments. Inhaling the steam from boiled cedar can help reduce fever and alleviate symptoms of chest colds and the flu. Sage, with its antimicrobial properties, has been traditionally used to treat wounds and prevent infections. Its leaves can be crushed and applied directly to the skin or brewed into a tea for internal use. Sweetgrass, often used as a mild sedative, helps to relax the mind and body. Its calming effects make it useful in treating anxiety and promoting restful sleep.

When sourcing and preparing these sacred herbs, it is crucial to follow sustainable and respectful practices. Ethical harvesting ensures that these plants continue to thrive for future generations.

Always seek permission from the land and take only what you need, leaving enough for the plant to regenerate. Drying and storing methods are essential for maintaining the potency of the herbs. Hang bundles of sage, sweetgrass, and cedar in a dry, dark place, allowing them to air dry slowly. Once dried, store them in airtight containers away from direct sunlight.

Creating smudge sticks and herbal bundles is a practical way to use these herbs in your daily rituals. For a sage smudge stick, gather fresh sage leaves and bind them tightly with natural twine. Allow the bundle to dry completely before using it for smudging. Sweetgrass can be braided while fresh and then dried, preserving its sweet aroma. Cedar branches can be bundled and hung to dry, ready to be used in both spiritual and medicinal applications.

Traditional recipes and rituals involving these sacred herbs offer a deep connection to Native American healing practices. To make a cedar tea, collect fresh cedar branches, place them in a pot of water, and bring to a boil. Simmer for about ten minutes until the water turns golden, and the aroma fills your home. Strain the liquid and sweeten it with honey or maple syrup if desired. Sweetgrass braiding is an art in itself. Divide the fresh grass into three sections and braid them together, focusing your intentions on peace and positivity. This braid can be used in ceremonies or hung in your home to invite good spirits.

PREPARING HERBAL TEAS FOR COMMON AILMENTS

When addressing common ailments, herbal teas have always been a cornerstone of Native American medicine. These teas are more than just comforting beverages; they are potent remedies designed to alleviate a variety of health issues. For instance, cold and flu symptoms are often treated with herbal teas that boost the immune system and soothe the respiratory tract. Digestive problems like indigestion, bloating, and cramps can be eased with the right blend of herbs. Anxiety and stress, which plague many of us in today's fast-paced world, can also be managed with calming herbal infusions.

Certain herbs stand out for their effectiveness in treating these common ailments. Peppermint is a go-to for digestive relief. Its natural antispasmodic properties help to relax the muscles of the gastrointestinal tract, easing symptoms like bloating and cramps. Elderberry is another powerful herb renowned for its immune-boosting capabilities. Rich in antioxidants and vitamins, elderberry can help fend off colds and flu, making it a staple during the colder months. Chamomile, known for its calming effects, is perfect for reducing anxiety and promoting restful sleep. Its gentle sedative properties make it ideal for winding down after a stressful day.

Preparing herbal teas at home is a straightforward process, yet it requires attention to detail to ensure you capture the full benefits of the herbs. Start by measuring your herbs accurately. A general rule of thumb is to use about one teaspoon of dried herbs or one tablespoon of fresh herbs per cup of water. Bring water to a boil, then pour it over the herbs in a teapot or mug. Cover the vessel to prevent the volatile oils from escaping, and let the tea steep for about 10-15 minutes. Strain the herbs out before drinking. Combining multiple herbs can create a synergistic effect, enhancing the overall efficacy of the tea. For instance, mixing peppermint with ginger not only aids digestion but also adds a warming, soothing element.

A cold and flu relief tea can be made using elderberry and echinacea. Both herbs are known for their immune-supporting properties. To prepare:

1. Combine one teaspoon of dried elderberries and one teaspoon of dried echinacea root in a teapot.
2. Add two cups of boiling water, cover, and let steep for 15 minutes.
3. Strain and sweeten with honey if desired.

This tea not only helps to ward off infections but also soothes the throat and reduces inflammation.

For digestive issues, a tea made with peppermint and ginger is highly effective. Peppermint alleviates bloating and gas, while ginger reduces nausea and stimulates digestion. Combine one teaspoon of dried peppermint leaves and one teaspoon of fresh, grated ginger in a teapot. Pour in two cups of boiling water, cover, and steep for 10 minutes. Strain and enjoy this soothing blend after meals to aid digestion and relieve discomfort.

A calming tea blend featuring chamomile and lavender can work wonders for anxiety and stress. Chamomile's gentle sedative effects and lavender's soothing aroma create a powerful relaxation aid. To prepare:

1. Mix one teaspoon of dried chamomile flowers and half a teaspoon of dried lavender buds in a teapot.
2. Add two cups of boiling water, cover, and steep for 10-15 minutes.
3. Strain and sip this fragrant tea in the evening to help unwind and prepare for a restful night's sleep.

Herbal teas offer a simple yet effective way to incorporate the healing power of Native American herbs into your daily routine. By understanding the properties of these herbs and mastering the preparation techniques, you can create personalized remedies that address your specific needs. Whether battling a cold, struggling with digestive issues, or seeking to reduce stress, an herbal tea blend can support your well-being.

CRAFTING SALVES AND OINTMENTS FROM NATIVE PLANTS

Salves and ointments are invaluable tools in any natural medicine cabinet. These topical remedies offer effective relief for a variety of conditions. Skin irritations and wounds, for instance, benefit immensely from the soothing and healing properties of certain herbs. A well-crafted salve can ease the discomfort of rashes, insect bites, and minor cuts. Muscle aches and joint pain are other ailments that respond well to herbal ointments. Specific plants' anti-inflammatory and analgesic properties penetrate the skin, providing targeted relief to sore muscles and arthritic joints. Burns, whether from the sun or minor kitchen accidents, also find comfort in the cooling and healing embrace of these herbal preparations.

Key native plants play a crucial role in the effectiveness of salves and ointments. Calendula, known for its bright orange and yellow flowers, is a powerhouse of anti-inflammatory and healing properties. It has been traditionally used to treat various skin conditions, from eczema to minor wounds, promoting faster healing and reducing inflammation. Arnica, a staple in many first-aid kits, is renowned for relieving pain and reducing bruising. Its application can swiftly ease the pain of sprains, strains, and contusions, making it an essential component in pain relief ointments. Plantain, often considered a common weed, is a remarkable herb for soothing skin irritations. Its leaves contain allantoin, a compound that encourages cell growth and accelerates the healing of damaged tissues.

Making your own salves and ointments at home is a rewarding process that ensures you know exactly what goes into your remedies. Begin by infusing oils with your chosen medicinal herbs. This step involves placing dried herbs in a jar and covering them with a carrier oil such as olive, coconut, or almond oil. Seal the jar and let it sit in a warm, sunny spot for several weeks, shaking it daily to encourage the extraction of the herb's active compounds. Once your oil is infused, strain out the plant material, and you're left with a potent herbal oil ready for the next step.

Combining your infused oil with beeswax is the key to achieving the right consistency for your salve or ointment. Beeswax not only thickens the oil but also adds protective and moisturizing properties. In a double boiler, gently heat your infused oil and beeswax together until the wax melts completely. The general ratio is one part beeswax to four parts oil, but you can adjust this based on your desired firmness. Once melted, remove from heat and stir in any essential oils for added benefits and fragrance. Essential oils like lavender, tea tree, or peppermint can enhance the therapeutic properties of your salve.

To create a healing salve with calendula and plantain, start with one cup of calendula-infused oil and one cup of plantain-infused oil. Combine these oils with half a cup of beeswax in a double boiler. Heat until the beeswax melts, then add 20 drops of lavender essential oil for its additional soothing effects. Pour the mixture into small jars and let it cool and solidify. This salve can be applied to cuts, scrapes, and irritated skin to promote healing and reduce inflammation.

For a pain-relief ointment using arnica and lavender, use one cup of arnica-infused oil and one cup of comfrey-infused oil. Combine these oils with half a cup of beeswax in a double boiler. Once the beeswax has melted, add 15 drops of lavender essential oil and 10 drops of peppermint essential oil for their analgesic properties. Stir well and pour into jars. This ointment is perfect for massaging into sore muscles and joints, providing relief from pain and inflammation.

A soothing balm for burns can be made with aloe vera and chamomile. Start with one cup of aloe vera gel and one cup of chamomile-infused oil. Heat the chamomile oil and half a cup of beeswax in a double boiler until the wax melts. Remove from heat and stir in the aloe vera gel and 20 drops of lavender essential oil. Pour into jars and allow to cool. This balm offers immediate relief from burns and helps to speed up the healing process while reducing pain and inflammation.

TRADITIONAL REMEDIES FOR RESPIRATORY HEALTH

Respiratory ailments have long been a challenge, but Native American remedies provide a natural approach to relief. Coughs and colds, for instance, are common issues that can be effectively managed with the right herbs. Asthma and bronchitis, conditions that cause inflammation and difficulty breathing, also benefit from these traditional practices. Allergies and sinus congestion, which can make daily life uncomfortable, are other areas where these remedies shine.

Mullein is particularly valued for its ability to soothe the respiratory tract. This tall, flowering plant has leaves that, when brewed into a tea, can help reduce inflammation and ease the symptoms of a cough or cold. The leaves and flowers contain compounds that act as natural expectorants, helping to clear mucus from the lungs.

Eucalyptus, known for its potent decongestant properties, is another key herb. The essential oil from eucalyptus leaves can open up nasal passages and ease breathing. Licorice root, with its anti-inflammatory effects, is often used to calm irritated airways. This sweet-tasting root reduces inflammation and helps protect the mucous membranes of the respiratory system.

Preparing and using these herbs for respiratory relief is straightforward and can be quite effective. Herbal steams and inhalations are a simple yet powerful method. Boil water and add a few drops of eucalyptus essential oil or a handful of fresh or dried eucalyptus leaves. Lean over the steaming pot with a towel draped over your head to trap the steam, and inhale deeply. This helps open up nasal passages and soothe the respiratory tract. Syrups and lozenges are another effective method. Mullein and licorice root can be simmered in water to create a concentrated decoction, which is then mixed with honey to make a soothing syrup. This can be taken by a spoonful several times a day to ease coughing and throat irritation. Herbal teas and infusions are also beneficial. Simply steeping mullein, licorice root, or eucalyptus in hot water can create a soothing drink that helps to ease respiratory discomfort.

For an herbal steam with eucalyptus and peppermint, boil a pot of water and add a handful of eucalyptus leaves and a few drops of peppermint essential oil. Lean over the pot with a towel over your head to trap the steam, and inhale deeply for about 10 minutes. This combination helps to clear nasal congestion and soothe the airways. Cough syrup with mullein and honey can be made by simmering two cups of mullein leaves in four cups of water until the liquid reduces by half. Strain the liquid and mix it with a cup of honey. Take a tablespoon of this syrup as needed to soothe a cough and reduce throat irritation. For a respiratory relief tea with licorice root and ginger, combine one teaspoon of dried licorice root with one teaspoon of freshly grated ginger in a teapot. Add two cups of boiling water, cover, and let steep for 10-15 minutes. Strain and drink this warming tea to help reduce inflammation and ease breathing.

These traditional remedies offer a natural and effective way to manage respiratory health. By understanding the properties of these herbs and learning how to prepare them, you can create your own personalized treatments for common respiratory issues. Whether you're dealing with a persistent cough, asthma, or seasonal allergies, these remedies provide a holistic approach to respiratory wellness.

THE USE OF PLANTS IN NATIVE AMERICAN RITUALS

Plants hold a profound spiritual significance in Native American rituals, serving as conduits between the physical and spiritual realms. These plants are more than just botanical entities; they are revered as sacred beings with their own spirits and energies. Sage, for instance, is frequently used in smudging ceremonies. This practice involves burning sage to produce smoke, which is believed to cleanse spaces, objects, and individuals of negative energies. The act of smudging is not just a physical process but a spiritual one, aiming to restore balance and harmony. As the smoke rises, it carries away impurities, creating a purified environment ready for positive energy and blessings.

Tobacco, another sacred plant, is often used in offerings and prayers. Unlike its recreational use in Native American traditions, tobacco is considered a powerful spiritual tool. It is offered to the spirits as a sign of respect and gratitude, facilitating communication with the divine. During ceremonies, small amounts of tobacco are placed in a fire, its smoke carrying prayers to the heavens. This act of offering tobacco is deeply symbolic, reflecting a connection with the spiritual world and seeking guidance and protection from the ancestors and spirits.

Sweetgrass, known for its sweet aroma, is integral to healing rituals. Often braided and burned, sweetgrass is believed to attract positive energies and good spirits. It is used to create a welcoming and harmonious atmosphere, both in personal spaces and during communal ceremonies. The scent of sweetgrass is considered soothing and uplifting, helping to alleviate stress and promote emotional healing. In many Native American cultures, sweetgrass is also used to bless new ventures, ensuring they begin with positive energy and intentions.

Specific rituals involving these sacred plants serve various spiritual and healing purposes. Smudging, for example, is performed to cleanse and purify. To properly smudge a space or person, first light the end of a sage bundle until it smolders, producing a steady stream of smoke. Hold the bundle over a fireproof bowl to catch any ashes. Use a feather or your hand to waft the smoke into the corners of the room, around objects, or over the person you are cleansing. As you do this, focus on your intention to clear away negative energy and invite positive forces.

Creating and offering a tobacco tie is another meaningful ritual. To make a tobacco tie, cut a small square of natural cloth, place a pinch of tobacco in the center, and gather the corners together, tying it with a natural string. Hold the tobacco tie in your hands and offer a prayer or set an intention. You can then place the tie in a special location, such as near a sacred fire or on an altar, as a physical representation of your offering and prayer.

Preparing and using a sweetgrass braid in rituals is a beautiful and fragrant practice. To braid sweetgrass, start by gathering three long strands of fresh sweetgrass. Tie them together at one end and begin braiding, focusing your mind on positive thoughts and intentions. Once braided, the sweetgrass can be dried and used in ceremonies. To use it, light one end of the braid until it smolders and produces smoke. Move the braid around the space or over a person, allowing the sweet aroma to fill the air and attract positive energies.

Respecting the cultural and ethical considerations of these practices is crucial. Understanding the cultural context of rituals is essential to honoring and preserving Native American traditions. These practices are deeply rooted in specific cultural beliefs and histories, and using them respectfully means acknowledging and valuing their origins. Ethical sourcing of sacred plants is also vital. Overharvesting and commercial exploitation can threaten these plants and the ecosystems they belong to. Always seek to source plants sustainably, taking only what you need and ensuring the plants can regenerate.

Seeking guidance from indigenous communities is another important step. Native American elders and healers possess the traditional knowledge and wisdom that can enrich your understanding and practice of these rituals. Building respectful relationships with these communities and learning from them directly can provide deeper insights and ensure that your practices are aligned with their cultural values and traditions. This approach not only honors the source of these sacred practices but also fosters cross-cultural understanding and respect.

HERBAL INFUSIONS FOR DIGESTIVE WELLNESS

Digestive issues can affect anyone, disrupting daily life and overall well-being. Common ailments like indigestion and bloating can cause significant discomfort. Indigestion, often accompanied by a feeling of fullness and gas, can make even the simplest meal a source of distress. Bloating, which results in a swollen abdomen, often occurs after eating and can be quite uncomfortable. Constipation and diarrhea represent opposite ends of the digestive spectrum, each with its own set of challenges. Constipation leads to infrequent, hard, and painful bowel movements, while diarrhea results in frequent, loose stools that can cause dehydration and nutritional deficiencies. Stomach cramps and nausea are other frequent complaints, often linked to digestive upset or stress. These issues can be particularly distressing, affecting appetite and daily activities.

Several herbs stand out for their effectiveness in supporting digestive health. Peppermint is a well-known ally for soothing the digestive tract. Its antispasmodic properties help relax the muscles of the gastrointestinal system, reducing symptoms of indigestion and bloating. The menthol in peppermint also has a cooling effect, which can be particularly comforting when dealing with digestive discomfort. Ginger is another powerhouse for digestive wellness. It's known for its ability to relieve nausea and stomach cramps; ginger stimulates digestive juices and enhances the movement of food through the digestive tract. This makes it an excellent remedy for both mild and severe digestive issues. Fennel, with its distinctive licorice-like flavor, is highly effective in reducing bloating and gas. Fennel seeds contain compounds that relax the smooth muscles of the gastrointestinal tract, allowing for the release of trapped gas and easing bloating.

Preparing herbal infusions for digestive wellness is a simple yet effective way to harness the healing power of these herbs. Start by measuring the herbs accurately to ensure proper dosage. A general guideline is to use about one teaspoon of dried herbs or one tablespoon of fresh herbs per cup of water. Bring the water to a boil, then pour it over the herbs in a teapot or mug. Cover the vessel to trap the essential oils and steep for about 10-15 minutes. Strain the herbs before drinking. Combining multiple herbs can enhance the overall effect of the infusion. For instance, mixing peppermint and fennel can provide a comprehensive remedy for indigestion and bloating, while combining ginger and chamomile offers both digestive and calming benefits.

For a soothing indigestion relief infusion, combine one teaspoon of dried peppermint leaves and one teaspoon of fennel seeds. Place the herbs in a teapot and pour in two cups of boiling water. Cover and steep for 10-15 minutes, then strain and sip slowly. This infusion not only eases indigestion but also helps to relax the digestive tract, reducing bloating and discomfort. For nausea relief, an infusion of ginger and chamomile can be particularly effective. Combine one teaspoon of grated fresh ginger and one teaspoon of dried chamomile flowers in a teapot. Add two cups of boiling water, cover, and steep for 15 minutes. Strain and drink this infusion to soothe nausea and calm the stomach. The warming properties of ginger combined with the calming effects of chamomile make this a powerful remedy for digestive upset.

To tackle bloating, an infusion with fennel and dandelion root is highly beneficial. Fennel helps to release trapped gas, while dandelion root acts as a gentle diuretic, reducing water retention that can contribute to bloating. Combine one teaspoon of fennel seeds and one teaspoon of dried dandelion root in a teapot. Pour in two cups of boiling water, cover, and steep for 10-15 minutes. Strain and drink to reduce bloating and support overall digestive health. This infusion not only eases immediate discomfort but also supports long-term digestive wellness by promoting healthy digestion and reducing water retention.

Herbal infusions provide a natural and effective way to address a variety of digestive issues. By understanding the properties of these herbs and learning how to prepare them, you can create personalized remedies that support your digestive health. Whether you're dealing with indigestion, bloating, or nausea, these infusions offer a holistic approach to digestive wellness, promoting comfort and well-being in your daily life.

In the next chapter, we will explore the rich traditions of Traditional Chinese Medicine, delving into its unique diagnostic methods and powerful herbal remedies.

CHAPTER 3: TRADITIONAL CHINESE MEDICINE REMEDIES

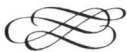

The first time I walked into a traditional Chinese medicine (TCM) shop, I was struck by the earthy, aromatic scents that filled the air. Rows of wooden drawers lined the walls, each labeled with Chinese characters, containing herbs I had never heard of but felt an immediate curiosity about. The shopkeeper, an elderly man with a serene demeanor, noticed my intrigue and began to explain the significance of some of the herbs. It was a moment of revelation, opening my eyes to the profound wisdom and centuries-old practices of TCM. This chapter delves into some of the most significant herbs in TCM, exploring their historical importance, medicinal properties, and practical uses.

KEY HERBS IN TRADITIONAL CHINESE MEDICINE

Ginseng, known as Ren Shen in Chinese, is one of the most revered herbs in TCM. Historically, it has been used for thousands of years to enhance vitality and energy. Ginseng is considered an adaptogen, meaning it helps the body adapt to stress and maintain balance. Its roots contain ginsenosides, active compounds that offer a range of health benefits. Ginseng is renowned for boosting both physical and mental performance. It enhances stamina, reduces fatigue, and improves cognitive function. Studies have shown that ginseng can improve physical endurance and mental sharpness, making it a popular choice for those seeking to enhance their overall well-being.

Astragalus, or Huang Qi, is another cornerstone of TCM. This herb is primarily known for its immune-boosting properties. It has been used to fortify the body's defenses against illnesses and to promote overall health. Astragalus contains polysaccharides and flavonoids, which have been shown to enhance immune function. Research supports its role in increasing the production of white blood cells, thereby helping the body fend off infections. Astragalus also has anti-inflammatory and antioxidant properties, making it a valuable herb for reducing oxidative stress and supporting long-term health.

Goji Berries, or Gou Qi Zi, are small red fruits packed with nutrients. They have been used in TCM for centuries to promote eye health and anti-aging. These berries are rich in antioxidants, particularly zeaxanthin, which helps protect the eyes from damage caused by free radicals. Goji berries are also known for their ability to improve skin health, boost immune function, and enhance overall vitality. Studies have indicated that regular consumption of goji berries can improve vision and reduce the risk of age-related eye conditions. Their anti-oxidative properties make them a popular choice for those looking to maintain a youthful appearance.

Licorice Root, known as Gan Cao, is often used as a harmonizer in herbal formulas. It helps to balance the effects of other herbs and enhances their overall efficacy. Licorice root has anti-inflammatory, antibacterial, and antiviral properties. It is commonly used to soothe sore throats, relieve digestive issues, and reduce inflammation. Licorice root is also known for its ability to modulate the immune system, making it helpful in treating various conditions. Its sweet flavor makes it a pleasant addition to herbal teas and remedies, and its harmonizing properties ensure that the other herbs in a formula work synergistically.

Scientific research has validated many of the traditional uses of these herbs. For instance, studies on ginseng have demonstrated its adaptogenic effects, showing that it helps the body maintain homeostasis under stress. Ginsenosides, the active compounds in ginseng, have been found to modulate the immune system, reduce inflammation, and improve cardiovascular health. Research on Astragalus has highlighted its impact on immune cells, showing that it enhances the activity of macrophages and natural killer cells, which are crucial for immune defense. Clinical trials on goji berries have shown their effectiveness in reducing oxidative stress and improving eye health, supporting their traditional use as a tonic for longevity and vitality.

When sourcing these herbs, it is crucial to find reputable suppliers who offer high-quality products. Look for suppliers who provide transparency about their sourcing practices and offer organic or sustainably harvested herbs. Proper drying and storing methods are essential to maintain the potency of the herbs. For example, ginseng roots should be dried slowly to preserve their active compounds and stored in airtight containers away from light and moisture. Simple preparation techniques can make these herbs a part of your daily routine. Ginseng can be sliced and brewed into tea, astragalus can be added to soups, and goji berries can be eaten as a snack or added to cereals and smoothies.

By understanding the historical significance, medicinal properties, and practical uses of these key herbs, you can integrate the wisdom of Traditional Chinese Medicine into your daily life. These herbs offer a natural and effective way to enhance your health and well-being, providing a holistic approach to modern health challenges.

PREPARING DECOCTIONS FOR IMMUNE SUPPORT

Herbal decoctions are a cornerstone of Traditional Chinese Medicine (TCM), valued for their ability to extract the full medicinal potential of herbs. Decoctions involve simmering herbs in water for an extended period, allowing the active compounds to be released and concentrated. This method is particularly effective for tough plant materials like roots, barks, and seeds, which require more time to break down and release their beneficial properties. Decoctions are favored over other forms of herbal preparations because they offer a potent and readily absorbable form of medicine. In TCM, decoctions are commonly used for their enhanced efficacy in treating various conditions, especially when a strong therapeutic effect is needed.

For immune support, certain herbs are frequently used in TCM decoctions due to their powerful properties. Astragalus, known as Huang Qi, is renowned for its ability to boost the immune system. It enhances the body's resistance to infections and helps to maintain overall health. Reishi Mushroom, or Ling Zhi, is another key herb. It is known for its immune-modulating effects and ability to enhance the body's resilience against illnesses. Isatis Root, called Ban Lan Gen, is traditionally used for its antiviral properties and is particularly effective in fighting off infections and supporting immune function.

Preparing herbal decoctions at home requires careful attention to measurement, dosage, and technique. Start by measuring the herbs accurately. A common ratio is to use about 10-15 grams of dried herbs per dose. Rinse the herbs under running water to remove any impurities, then soak them in clean water for about 30 minutes to soften them. This step helps to prepare the herbs for the simmering process. Place the soaked herbs in a ceramic pot, as ceramic is chemically stable and provides even heat transmission, ensuring that the herbs are decocted properly. Add enough water to cover the herbs by about 2-3 centimeters.

Bring the water to a boil, then reduce the heat to a gentle simmer. Allow the herbs to simmer for 30-45 minutes, stirring occasionally to ensure even extraction. This slow simmering process is crucial for extracting the medicinal compounds from the herbs. Once the decoction is ready, strain the liquid into a clean container, discarding the spent herbs. The resulting liquid is your herbal decoction, a concentrated form of herbal medicine ready for use. For enhanced effects, you can combine multiple herbs in a single decoction, allowing their properties to work synergistically.

To make an immune-boosting decoction with Astragalus and Reishi Mushroom:

1. Start with 15 grams of dried Astragalus root and 10 grams of dried Reishi Mushroom slices.
2. Rinse and soak the herbs, then place them in a ceramic pot with enough water to cover them.
3. Bring to a boil, reduce to a simmer, and let it cook for 45 minutes.
4. Strain the liquid and drink it warm.

This decoction enhances immune function and supports overall vitality and resilience.

For an antiviral decoction, combine 10 grams of Isatis Root with 10 grams of Forsythia. These herbs are known for their strong antiviral properties and are particularly effective during cold and flu season. Rinse and soak the herbs, then simmer them in a ceramic pot for 30 minutes. Strain and drink the decoction warm. This preparation helps to fend off viral infections and supports the body's natural defenses.

A general immune support decoction can be made using a blend of multiple herbs for a comprehensive effect. Combine 10 grams of Astragalus, 10 grams of Reishi Mushroom, and 5 grams of Isatis Root. Rinse and soak the herbs, then simmer them together for 45 minutes. Strain the liquid and drink it warm. This multi-herb decoction provides a robust boost to the immune system, enhancing the body's ability to resist infections and maintain health.

By understanding the process of making herbal decoctions and the benefits of key immune-supporting herbs, you can create powerful, natural remedies to enhance your immune system. Decoctions offer a potent and effective way to integrate the wisdom of Traditional Chinese Medicine into your daily health routine, providing a holistic approach to maintaining wellness and resilience.

HERBAL REMEDIES FOR STRESS AND ANXIETY

In the hustle and bustle of modern life, managing stress and anxiety has become a priority for many. Traditional Chinese Medicine (TCM) offers a nuanced approach to emotional well-being, rooted in the principles of Qi and the balance of Yin and Yang. Qi, the vital energy that flows through the body, can become stagnant due to stress, leading to emotional and physical symptoms. This stagnation disrupts the harmonious flow of energy, contributing to feelings of anxiety and tension. Balancing Yin and Yang is essential for maintaining emotional equilibrium. When Yin and Yang are out of balance, it can manifest as heightened stress or anxiety. TCM employs herbs to restore this balance, helping the body and mind cope with stress more effectively.

Adaptogens play a significant role in this process. These are herbs that help the body adapt to stress by modulating the release of stress hormones and supporting the adrenal glands. They work by normalizing bodily functions, providing a calming effect without sedation. Adaptogens are particularly useful because they help the body maintain homeostasis, making it more resilient to stressors. This adaptability is crucial for emotional well-being, as it allows the body to handle the ups and downs of life better.

Several key herbs in TCM are renowned for their ability to alleviate stress and anxiety. Suan Zao Ren, or Ziziphus Seed, is a staple in TCM for calming the mind. It is often used to treat insomnia and anxiety, helping to stabilize mood and promote restful sleep. The seeds contain compounds that soothe the nervous system, making them effective in reducing stress. Bai He, known as Lily Bulb, nourishes the heart and calms the spirit. It is particularly beneficial for those experiencing emotional turmoil and heart palpitations. The herb's gentle effects help to ease anxiety and support overall emotional health. Long Gu, or Dragon Bone, is used for grounding and stabilizing emotions. This mineral-rich herb is often prescribed for severe anxiety and restlessness, providing a sense of calm and stability.

Preparing and using these herbs for stress relief can be both simple and effective. Herbal teas and infusions are a popular method. To make a calming tea, combine Suan Zao Ren and Bai He. Measure one teaspoon of each herb and steep them in hot water for about 15 minutes. This tea can be consumed in the evening to promote relaxation and improve sleep quality. Tinctures and extracts offer a more concentrated form of these herbs. To prepare a stress-relief tincture, combine Dragon Bone and Schisandra. Use a 1:5 ratio of herbs to alcohol, such as vodka or brandy. Allow the mixture to macerate for several weeks, shaking it daily. Strain the liquid into a dark glass bottle and take a few drops as needed to alleviate anxiety.

Creating herbal baths and soaks is another soothing way to incorporate these herbs into your routine. A herbal bath with Lavender and Chamomile can provide immediate relief from stress. Add a handful of dried lavender flowers and chamomile to a muslin bag and place it in your bathwater. Soak for at least 20 minutes, allowing the herbs to infuse the water and your skin to absorb their calming properties. This practice not only relaxes the body but also calms the mind, creating a serene environment for stress relief.

For a specific stress-relief recipe, consider making a calming tea with Ziziphu Seeds and a Lily Bulb. Combine one teaspoon of Suan Zao Ren and one teaspoon of Bai He in a teapot. Pour in two cups of boiling water, cover, and let steep for 15 minutes. Strain the herbs and sip the tea slowly in the evening. This blend not only calms the mind but also nourishes the heart, providing a holistic approach to stress relief. Another effective recipe is a stress-relief tincture with Dragon Bone and Schisandra. Use 10 grams of Dragon Bone and 10 grams of Schisandra berries. Place the herbs in a glass jar and cover with 100 milliliters of alcohol. Let the mixture steep for four weeks, shaking it daily. Strain and store in a dark bottle. Take a few drops under the tongue during times of high stress.

Creating a herbal bath with Lavender and Chamomile is simple yet effective. Fill a muslin bag with equal parts dried lavender flowers and chamomile. Tie the bag securely and place it in your bathwater. Allow it to steep as you fill the tub, then soak for at least 20 minutes. The soothing aroma and therapeutic properties of these herbs help to relieve stress and promote relaxation, making it an ideal way to unwind after a long day.

By integrating these TCM herbs into your routine, you can effectively manage stress and anxiety. These natural remedies offer a holistic approach to emotional well-being, helping you to find balance and tranquility in your daily life. Whether through teas, tinctures, or baths, these practices provide simple yet powerful tools for enhancing your mental and emotional health.

CRAFTING TINCTURES FOR LONGEVITY AND VITALITY

Tinctures are a favored method in Traditional Chinese Medicine (TCM) for their potency and convenience. These concentrated herbal extracts capture the essence of the herbs, making them highly effective. The process of creating tinctures involves soaking herbs in alcohol, which extracts and preserves their active compounds. This results in a potent solution that is easy to use and has a long shelf life. Unlike teas or decoctions, tinctures are quick to take, requiring just a few drops under the tongue or diluted in water. Their small size makes them portable, allowing you to maintain your health routine effortlessly.

He Shou Wu, also known as Fo-Ti, is a key herb in TCM tinctures for longevity and vitality. Traditionally used for its anti-aging properties, He Shou Wu is believed to promote hair health and restore youthful vigor. Reishi Mushroom, a revered herb in TCM, is another excellent choice for tinctures. Known for its immune-supporting and longevity-promoting effects, Reishi Mushroom helps enhance the body's resilience and overall well-being. Ginseng, celebrated for its energy-boosting properties, is a staple in vitality tinctures. This adaptogenic herb not only increases physical stamina but also supports mental clarity and focus.

Creating tinctures at home begins with selecting the right herbs and alcohol base. Choose high-quality dried or fresh herbs from reputable suppliers to ensure potency. For the alcohol base, use a high-proof vodka or brandy, as these effectively extract the medicinal compounds from the herbs. Measure the herbs accurately; a general guideline is one part herb to five parts alcohol by volume. Place the herbs in a clean, dry glass jar and cover them with alcohol, ensuring the herbs are fully submerged. Seal the jar tightly and store it in a cool, dark place. Shake the jar daily to encourage extraction and prevent the herbs from settling.

The maceration process typically takes four to six weeks. This allows the alcohol to extract the active compounds from the herbs thoroughly. After the maceration period:

1. Strain the mixture through a fine mesh strainer or cheesecloth into another clean jar.
2. Squeeze out as much liquid as possible from the herbs to ensure you capture all the medicinal properties.
3. Pour the strained liquid into dark glass bottles with droppers for easy use.
4. Label the bottles with the contents and date of preparation.

For an anti-aging tincture with Fo-Ti and Goji Berries, combine 50 grams of dried Fo-Ti root with 50 grams of dried Goji Berries. Place the herbs in a glass jar and cover with 500 milliliters of vodka. Seal the jar and store it in a cool, dark place for six weeks, shaking it daily. After six weeks, strain the liquid into dark glass bottles. Take one to two droppers full daily to support longevity and vitality.

A vitality tincture with Ginseng and Astragalus can be made by combining 50 grams of dried Ginseng root with 50 grams of dried

Astragalus root. Place the herbs in a jar and cover with 500 milliliters of brandy. Seal and store in a cool, dark place, shaking daily for six weeks. Strain and bottle the tincture. This blend enhances energy and supports overall well-being. Take one to two droppers full as needed, especially during periods of physical or mental exertion.

For an immune-boosting tincture with Reishi and Licorice Root, combine 50 grams of dried Reishi Mushroom slices with 50 grams of dried Licorice Root. Place the herbs in a jar and cover with 500 milliliters of vodka. Seal the jar and store it in a cool, dark place, shaking it daily for six weeks. Strain the tincture into dark glass bottles. This blend supports the immune system and enhances resilience. Take one to two droppers full daily, particularly during cold and flu season or times of increased stress.

By crafting tinctures with these powerful herbs, you can harness the wisdom of Traditional Chinese Medicine to promote longevity and vitality. These tinctures offer a convenient and effective way to integrate herbal medicine into your daily routine, supporting a healthier and more vibrant life.

THE ROLE OF ADAPTOGENS IN CHINESE MEDICINE

Adaptogens are a fascinating group of herbs that help the body adapt to various forms of stress, maintaining balance and promoting overall well-being. In Traditional Chinese Medicine (TCM), the concept of adaptogens has been integral for centuries. These herbs are known for their ability to enhance the body's resilience, making it easier to cope with physical, emotional, and environmental stressors. Historically, adaptogens have been used in TCM to support longevity and vitality, ensuring that the body remains in a state of harmony regardless of external pressures. Modern scientific research has validated many of these traditional uses, showing that adaptogens can indeed modulate stress responses, improve energy levels, and support immune function.

One of the most important adaptogenic herbs in TCM is Ginseng, which is prized for boosting energy and enhancing stress resistance. Ginseng contains active compounds called ginsenosides, which help to regulate the body's stress response by modulating the release of stress hormones. This herb is particularly effective in improving physical stamina and mental clarity, making it a popular choice for those looking to enhance their overall performance. Schisandra is another key adaptogen in TCM. Known for its liver-supporting and endurance-boosting properties, Schisandra helps to detoxify the body and improve physical performance. It contains lignans and other compounds that support liver function and enhance the body's ability to withstand stress. Rhodiola, often referred to as the "golden root," is celebrated for its ability to reduce fatigue and improve mental clarity. This herb works by enhancing the production of neurotransmitters that regulate mood and energy levels, making it an excellent choice for combating stress and promoting emotional balance.

The benefits of adaptogens extend beyond stress resistance. They play a crucial role in enhancing both physical and mental performance. By modulating the release of stress hormones, adaptogens help to maintain optimal energy levels and improve cognitive function. This makes them particularly useful for those who face high levels of physical or mental exertion. Adaptogens also boost immune function by enhancing the activity of immune cells and reducing inflammation. This dual action not only helps the body fight off infections but also reduces the risk of chronic diseases. Additionally, adaptogens promote emotional balance by regulating neurotransmitter levels, helping to alleviate symptoms of anxiety and depression. Their calming effects make them a natural choice for those seeking to improve their emotional well-being.

Incorporating adaptogens into your daily life can be both simple and effective. One of the easiest ways to enjoy the benefits of adaptogens is by making teas and smoothies. For an adaptogenic tea, you can steep slices of dried Ginseng or a combination of Schisandra berries and Rhodiola root in hot water for about 10-15 minutes. This creates a potent brew that can help you start your day with increased energy and focus. Adding adaptogen powders to food is another convenient option. You can sprinkle powdered Ginseng or Schisandra into your morning oatmeal, yogurt, or smoothie. This not only enhances the nutritional value of your meals but also ensures a steady intake of these beneficial herbs.

Preparing adaptogenic tinctures and capsules offers another effective way to incorporate these herbs into your routine. Tinctures are particularly potent and easy to use. To make an adaptogenic tincture:

1. Combine equal parts of dried Ginseng, Schisandra, and Rhodiola in a glass jar and cover with high-proof vodka or brandy.
2. Seal the jar and store it in a cool, dark place for six weeks, shaking it daily.
3. After six weeks, strain the liquid into dark glass bottles. This tincture can be taken by the dropperful as needed to boost energy and reduce stress.

Capsules are another convenient form of adaptogens. You can purchase pre-made adaptogen capsules or make your own by filling empty gelatin capsules with powdered Ginseng, Schisandra, and Rhodiola. This method ensures that you get a consistent dose of adaptogens without the need for preparation.

By understanding the role of adaptogens in Chinese Medicine and learning how to incorporate them into your daily routine, you can harness their powerful benefits to improve your overall health and well-being. These herbs offer a natural and effective way to enhance your body's resilience, helping you to better manage stress and maintain balance in your life.

USING CHINESE HERBS IN DAILY DIETS

Incorporating Traditional Chinese Medicine (TCM) herbs into your daily meals can greatly enhance your nutritional intake and provide preventative health benefits. The principles of TCM dietary therapy emphasize the use of herbs to not only treat ailments but also to maintain overall health. By integrating these herbs into your everyday diet, you can enjoy their medicinal properties while also enhancing the flavors of your meals. This approach aligns with the TCM philosophy of prevention, where regular consumption of medicinal herbs helps to fortify the body against disease and maintain balance.

One of the most commonly used culinary herbs in TCM is ginger. It's known for its warming properties, and ginger helps stimulate digestion and improve circulation. It is often used in soups, teas, and stir-fries to add a zesty flavor while promoting digestive health. Garlic is another staple in TCM cooking. Its antimicrobial and immune-boosting effects make it an excellent addition to a variety of dishes. Garlic can help ward off infections and support overall immune function. Goji berries, with their rich antioxidant content, are frequently used in both sweet and savory dishes. These berries are known for their ability to promote eye health and provide anti-aging benefits. Adding them to your meals can boost your intake of essential nutrients and enhance your overall health.

A simple yet nourishing recipe that incorporates these herbs is a warming ginger and garlic soup. To make this soup:

1. Start by sautéing minced garlic and ginger in a pot with a bit of oil.
2. Add sliced mushrooms and continue to cook until they soften.
3. Pour in vegetable or chicken broth and bring to a simmer.
4. Add in some greens like bok choy or spinach, and let the soup cook until the greens are tender.
5. Season with a bit of soy sauce and serve hot.

This soup not only warms the body but also supports digestion and boosts immunity.

Another delightful recipe is Goji Berry and Red Date tea, which is excellent for daily health maintenance. To prepare this tea:

1. Combine a handful of dried goji berries and a few sliced red dates in a pot.
2. Add water and bring to a boil, then reduce to a simmer and let it cook for about 20 minutes.
3. Strain the tea and enjoy it warm.

This tea is rich in antioxidants and vitamins, making it a perfect drink to support your daily health routine.

For a more substantial meal, consider making a stir-fry with medicinal mushrooms and herbs. Start by heating some oil in a wok or large pan. Add sliced garlic and ginger, and stir-fry until fragrant. Add a mix of mushrooms such as shiitake, maitake, and reishi, and cook until they begin to soften. Toss in some greens and perhaps a protein like tofu or chicken. Season with soy sauce, a splash of rice vinegar, and a pinch of crushed red pepper for a bit of heat. Serve over steamed rice or noodles. This dish not only tastes delicious but also provides a wealth of nutrients and medicinal benefits.

The balance of flavors and energies in TCM meals is guided by the Five Flavors and their corresponding organs. These flavors—sweet, sour, bitter, salty, and pungent—each affect different organs and aspects of health. For instance, sweet flavors nourish the spleen, while sour flavors benefit the liver. Balancing warming and cooling foods is also crucial. Warming foods like ginger and garlic help to stimulate and energize the body, while cooling foods like cucumber and mint help to calm and detoxify. According to TCM principles, seasonal eating ensures that you are consuming foods that support your body's needs throughout the year.

For example, in the winter, warming and nourishing foods are emphasized to protect against the cold, while in the summer, cooling and hydrating foods are preferred to balance the heat.

In the next chapter, we will explore the rich traditions of ancient remedies from other cultures around the world, delving into their unique herbal practices and the wisdom they offer us today.

CHAPTER 4: GLOBAL ANCIENT REMEDIES

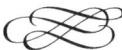

Walking through a bustling Indian spice market, I was instantly captivated by the vibrant colors and intoxicating scents of the myriad herbs and spices displayed in heaping mounds. The market was alive with the chatter of vendors and the hum of customers, each seeking remedies for various ailments or simply to enrich their daily lives. It was here that I first learned about Ayurveda, an ancient system of medicine that has been practiced for thousands of years. The wisdom contained in this traditional Indian practice is profound, offering natural solutions for modern health challenges.

AYURVEDIC HERBS AND THEIR HEALING PROPERTIES

Ayurveda, a holistic system of medicine from India, is guided by the principles of balance and harmony within the body. At the core of Ayurvedic medicine are the three doshas: Vata, Pitta, and Kapha. These doshas represent different combinations of the five basic elements—earth, water, fire, air, and ether—and each person has a unique constitution, or Prakriti, determined by the balance of these doshas. Vata, composed of air and ether, governs movement and communication. Pitta, made of fire and water, controls digestion and metabolism. Kapha, consisting of earth and water, is responsible for structure and lubrication. The goal of Ayurveda is to maintain balance among these doshas to achieve optimal health. An imbalance in any of the doshas can lead to physical and mental ailments, and Ayurvedic treatments aim to restore this harmony.

One of the most revered herbs in Ayurveda is Ashwagandha, known for its ability to reduce stress and enhance vitality. This adaptogenic herb helps the body cope with stress by modulating cortisol levels and supporting adrenal function. It also boosts energy, improves muscle strength, and enhances overall well-being. Turmeric, another cornerstone of Ayurvedic medicine, is celebrated for its powerful anti-inflammatory properties. The active compound in turmeric, curcumin, has been extensively studied for its ability to reduce inflammation, alleviate pain, and support joint health. Triphala, a traditional Ayurvedic blend of three fruits (Amalaki, Bibhitaki, and Haritaki), is renowned for its digestive benefits. It acts as a gentle laxative, stimulates appetite, and supports overall digestive health.

Preparing these Ayurvedic herbs involves various traditional methods that maximize their healing properties. Herbal teas and decoctions are commonly used to extract medicinal compounds from herbs. To make a simple Ashwagandha tea, you can simmer one teaspoon of Ashwagandha powder in a cup of water for about 10 minutes, strain, and drink. This tea helps reduce stress and promote relaxation. Herbal pastes and poultices are another method often used for topical applications. For example, a turmeric paste can be made by mixing turmeric powder with water or oil to create a thick paste, which can be applied to inflamed or painful areas to reduce inflammation and promote healing.

Ayurvedic massage, or Abhyanga, is an integral part of this traditional practice. It involves the use of warm herbal oils, which are massaged into the skin to nourish the body and mind. The oils are often infused with herbs like Ashwagandha and Turmeric to enhance their therapeutic effects. This practice not only supports physical health by improving circulation and detoxification but also promotes mental clarity and emotional balance.

For those interested in incorporating Ayurvedic practices into their daily routine, here are some specific recipes to get started. A calming Ashwagandha milk is an excellent evening drink to unwind and prepare for restful sleep. To make it, heat a cup of milk (or a plant-based alternative) and add one teaspoon of Ashwagandha powder, a pinch of nutmeg, and a sweetener like honey or maple syrup. Stir well and drink warm. This soothing beverage helps reduce stress and promotes relaxation.

A turmeric paste for inflammation can be easily prepared by mixing one tablespoon of turmeric powder with a bit of water or oil to form a thick paste. Apply this paste to inflamed joints or muscles and leave it on for 15-20 minutes before rinsing off. The anti-inflammatory properties of turmeric help reduce pain and swelling.

Triphala churna, a traditional Ayurvedic digestive aid, can be taken daily to support digestive health. Mix one teaspoon of Triphala powder with a glass of warm water and drink it before bed. This gentle laxative helps cleanse the digestive tract, stimulates the appetite, and supports overall digestive wellness.

Ayurveda offers a wealth of knowledge for anyone seeking natural and holistic health solutions. By understanding the principles of the three doshas and the importance of individual constitution, you can tailor Ayurvedic practices to meet your specific needs. Incorporating key Ayurvedic herbs like Ashwagandha, Turmeric, and Triphala into your daily routine through teas, pastes, and massages can significantly enhance your well-being. The recipes provided here are simple yet powerful, offering a practical introduction to the profound benefits of Ayurvedic medicine.

ANCIENT EGYPTIAN HERBAL PRACTICES

Ancient Egyptian civilization was a beacon of advanced knowledge in many fields, and medicine was no exception. Among the various medical texts that have survived, the Ebers Papyrus stands out. This extensive document, dating back to around 1550 BCE, is one of the oldest medical texts in existence. It details over 700 remedies and incantations, providing a glimpse into the sophisticated and holistic approach of ancient Egyptian medicine. The Ebers Papyrus highlights the integral role of priests and healers, who were often seen as intermediaries between the gods and the people. These practitioners combined their knowledge of herbs with spiritual practices, believing that magic and medicine were deeply intertwined. Healing rituals often included prayers and incantations to invoke divine assistance, reflecting a culture where the physical and spiritual realms were closely connected.

Among the many herbs used by ancient Egyptians, Aloe Vera was highly valued for its skin-healing properties. This succulent plant, with its thick, fleshy leaves, was used to treat burns, wounds, and various skin conditions. The gel inside the leaves contains compounds that promote healing and reduce inflammation. Frankincense, a resin obtained from the Boswellia tree, was another important herb. It was prized for its anti-inflammatory properties and used in both medicinal and ceremonial contexts. Frankincense was often burned as incense to purify spaces and was also applied as a paste to inflamed areas of the body. Myrrh, another resin, was renowned for its antiseptic and healing properties. It was used to treat wounds and prevent infections, and its aromatic qualities made it a staple in religious rituals.

The preparation and use of these herbs in ancient Egypt were meticulous and thoughtful. Making ointments and salves was a common method to harness the healing properties of plants. Aloe Vera gel, for example, was often mixed with other ingredients to create soothing ointments for burns and wounds. To prepare an Aloe Vera ointment, the gel from the leaves was extracted and combined with animal fats or oils to create a smooth, spreadable mixture. This ointment was then applied directly to the skin to promote healing and reduce pain.

Herbal poultices and compresses were another traditional preparation method. These involved crushing or grinding herbs into a paste, which was then applied to the affected area and covered with a cloth. For instance, a poultice made from myrrh could be used to treat infected wounds. The antiseptic properties of myrrh helped to clean the wound and prevent further infection. Compresses soaked in herbal infusions were also used to reduce inflammation and soothe pain.

Creating incense and fumigants was a practice that combined the medicinal and spiritual uses of herbs. Frankincense and myrrh were often burned to produce aromatic smoke that was believed to purify the air and protect against disease. This smoke was inhaled or allowed to permeate living spaces, providing both a calming atmosphere and therapeutic benefits. The preparation of incense involved grinding the resins into a fine powder, which was then shaped into pellets or sticks for burning.

For those interested in experimenting with ancient Egyptian herbal practices, here are some specific recipes. An Aloe Vera ointment for skin healing can be made by mixing fresh Aloe Vera gel with a carrier oil, such as coconut or olive oil, and a small amount of beeswax to thicken the mixture. Heat the oil and beeswax together until melted, then stir in the Aloe Vera gel and allow the mixture to cool and solidify. This ointment can be applied to minor burns, cuts, and dry skin.

A Frankincense and Myrrh salve for wounds can be prepared by combining equal parts of frankincense and myrrh resins with a carrier oil and beeswax. Heat the oil and beeswax until melted, then stir in the powdered resins until fully incorporated. Pour the mixture into small containers and let it cool. This salve can be used to treat inflamed or infected wounds, providing both antiseptic and anti-inflammatory benefits.

To create an herbal incense for purification, grind equal parts of frankincense and myrrh resins into a fine powder. Mix the powders together and form small pellets or sticks. These can be burned on a charcoal disc or in an incense burner to produce a fragrant smoke that purifies the air and creates a calming atmosphere. This incense can be used in meditation, rituals, or simply to enhance the ambiance of your home.

TRADITIONAL AFRICAN PLANT REMEDIES

African herbal medicine is incredibly diverse, reflecting the continent's vast array of ecosystems and cultural practices. Traditional healers and herbalists hold a revered place in many African communities, acting as custodians of ancient wisdom and practitioners of both spiritual and medicinal healing. These individuals are often seen as the bridge between the physical and spiritual realms, employing a holistic approach to health that encompasses the mind, body, and spirit. Spiritual practices are deeply integrated into medicinal treatments, with rituals and ceremonies often accompanying the use of herbs to enhance their efficacy. Regional variations in plant use and preparation methods are notable across the continent, from the savannas of West Africa to the rainforests of Central Africa, each region harnessing local flora to address specific health needs.

Devil's Claw, native to the arid regions of Southern Africa, is renowned for its potent anti-inflammatory and analgesic properties. Traditionally used to treat pain and inflammation, it has gained popularity in Western herbal medicine for its effectiveness in managing arthritis and other inflammatory conditions. The tubers of the plant are dried and ground into a powder, which can be used to make decoctions or incorporated into topical applications. Rooibos, hailing from South Africa, is another significant plant with powerful antioxidant properties. This red bush tea, caffeine-free and rich in polyphenols, supports overall health by neutralizing free radicals and reducing oxidative stress. African Ginger, known for its digestive benefits, is used to alleviate nausea, improve digestion, and soothe gastrointestinal discomfort. The rhizomes are often chewed raw or brewed into teas and infusions, providing a natural remedy for various digestive issues.

The preparation and usage of these plants are rooted in traditional practices that have been passed down through generations. Herbal infusions and decoctions are common methods for extracting the medicinal compounds from these plants. For example, a decoction of Devil's Claw can be prepared by simmering the dried, powdered tubers in water for about 15-20 minutes. This concentrated liquid can be consumed to alleviate pain and inflammation. Herbal poultices and compresses are also widely used, especially for topical treatments. To make a poultice with Devil's Claw, mix the powdered tubers with a small amount of water to form a paste. Apply this paste directly to the affected area and cover it with a clean cloth. This method allows the anti-inflammatory properties to penetrate the skin and provide localized relief.

Spiritual rituals and ceremonies often involve the use of these medicinal plants to enhance their healing effects. In many African cultures, the preparation and administration of herbal remedies are accompanied by prayers, chants, or offerings to the ancestors and spirits. These practices are believed to invoke spiritual support and ensure the effectiveness of the treatment. Rooibos, for instance, is often used in cleansing rituals where the tea is sprinkled around the home to purify the space and protect against negative energies. The aromatic steam from a Rooibos infusion can also be inhaled to clear the respiratory tract and promote relaxation.

For those interested in exploring African herbal remedies, here are some specific recipes. A pain relief balm with Devil's Claw can be made by blending the powdered tubers with a carrier oil, such as coconut or olive oil, and beeswax. Heat the oil and beeswax together until melted, then stir in the Devil's Claw powder until fully incorporated. Pour the mixture into small containers and let it cool. This balm can be applied to sore joints and muscles to reduce pain and inflammation.

To make a Rooibos tea for antioxidant support, simply steep one teaspoon of Rooibos leaves in a cup of boiling water for 5-7 minutes. Strain the leaves and enjoy the tea hot or cold. This refreshing beverage provides antioxidant benefits and supports overall health and well-being.

For a digestive aid infusion with African Ginger, slice a small piece of fresh ginger root and add it to a cup of boiling water. Let it steep for 10-15 minutes, then strain and drink the infusion. This simple yet effective remedy can help alleviate nausea, improve digestion, and soothe gastrointestinal discomfort.

African herbal medicine offers a rich tapestry of natural remedies that are deeply rooted in cultural traditions and practices. By understanding the diverse regional practices, key medicinal plants, and traditional preparation methods, you can appreciate the profound wisdom embedded in these ancient healing traditions. Incorporating these remedies into your daily routine can provide natural and effective solutions for various health issues, promoting overall well-being and a deeper connection to nature.

INDIGENOUS AUSTRALIAN BUSH MEDICINE

Indigenous Australian bush medicine is a profound testament to the deep connection between people and the land. These practices are steeped in cultural significance, with Dreamtime stories playing a pivotal role in understanding the uses of various plants. Dreamtime, the Aboriginal understanding of the world's creation, is not just a collection of myths but a living, breathing spiritual framework. These stories explain the origins of plants and animals and their roles in the ecosystem, guiding the use of flora for healing purposes. Elders and traditional healers, who are the custodians of this knowledge, play a crucial role in passing down these stories and practices through generations. Their wisdom integrates spiritual and physical healing, emphasizing that true health encompasses the mind, body, and spirit.

One of the most revered plants in Indigenous Australian medicine is the Tea Tree. It's known for its powerful antiseptic properties; Tea Tree oil is used to treat cuts, wounds, and infections. The oil, extracted from the leaves of the Melaleuca alternifolia tree, contains compounds that are effective against bacteria, viruses, and fungi. Eucalyptus is another vital plant, prized for its respiratory health benefits. The leaves of the Eucalyptus tree are rich in eucalyptol, a compound that works as a decongestant and anti-inflammatory agent, making it ideal for treating colds and respiratory infections. Kakadu Plum, a fruit native to northern Australia, boasts the highest natural vitamin C content of any plant in the world. This makes it an excellent immune booster and a valuable addition to the diet for overall health.

Traditionally, these plants are prepared and used in various ways to harness their medicinal properties. Herbal infusions and teas are commonly made by steeping the leaves or fruit in hot water to extract their beneficial compounds. For instance, a simple Tea Tree infusion can be made by boiling a handful of Tea Tree leaves in water, then straining the liquid and using it as a wash for wounds or skin infections. Poultices and topical applications are also prevalent. Crushed Eucalyptus leaves can be applied directly to the skin to relieve pain and inflammation or used in a steam inhalation to clear congested airways. Smoking ceremonies, where plants like Eucalyptus are burned to produce aromatic smoke, serve both spiritual and medicinal purposes, cleansing the environment and promoting respiratory health.

For those interested in trying bush medicine, an antiseptic wash with Tea Tree is a practical place to start. Boil a handful of Tea Tree leaves in water for about 10 minutes, strain, and let the liquid cool. This wash can be used to clean cuts, insect bites, and minor infections, harnessing the antibacterial properties of Tea Trees. A respiratory relief steam with Eucalyptus can be prepared by adding a few fresh or dried Eucalyptus leaves to a bowl of hot water. Lean over the bowl with a towel draped over your head to trap the steam, and inhale deeply for 10 minutes. This method helps to clear nasal passages and soothe respiratory discomfort.

An immune-boosting Kakadu Plum tonic is another valuable remedy. Simply blend fresh or dried Kakadu Plums with water to create a nutritious drink rich in vitamin C. This tonic can be consumed daily to enhance immune function and protect against illnesses. The high antioxidant content of Kakadu Plum also supports overall health, making it a powerful addition to your wellness routine.

Indigenous Australian bush medicine offers a rich and diverse array of natural remedies deeply rooted in cultural traditions and spiritual practices. By understanding the cultural significance, key medicinal plants, and traditional preparation methods, you can appreciate the depth and wisdom of these ancient healing practices. These remedies provide natural and effective solutions for various health issues, promoting holistic well-being and a deeper connection to the natural world.

SOUTH AMERICAN HERBAL HEALING TRADITIONS

Walking through the vibrant markets of South America, you're bound to encounter stalls brimming with an array of herbs, roots, and tinctures. These markets are a testament to the region's rich history of herbal medicine, deeply intertwined with the cultural practices of ancient civilizations like the Incas and Aztecs. These societies had a profound knowledge of plants and their healing properties, passed down through generations by shamans and traditional healers. Shamans, often regarded as spiritual leaders, played a crucial role in these communities. They used their extensive knowledge of herbal medicine in conjunction with spiritual practices to treat ailments, believing that physical health was closely linked to spiritual well-being.

One of the most revered plants in South American herbal medicine is Maca. Grown in the high Andes of Peru, Maca is known for its ability to boost energy and balance hormones. The root of the Maca plant is rich in vitamins, minerals, and amino acids, making it a powerful adaptogen that helps the body adapt to stress and maintain homeostasis. It's often used to enhance stamina, increase fertility, and alleviate symptoms of menopause. Another significant plant is Cat's Claw, a vine native to the Amazon rainforest. Cat's Claw is renowned for its immune-supporting properties. The bark and root of the plant contain compounds that boost the immune system, reduce inflammation, and protect against infections. Yerba Mate, a traditional South American tea, is famous for its stimulant properties. Made from the leaves of the Ilex paraguariensis plant, Yerba Mate is rich in antioxidants and caffeine, providing a natural energy boost and improving mental alertness.

Traditional preparation methods for these plants are designed to extract their maximum medicinal benefits. Herbal teas and infusions are a common way to consume these plants. To make a Maca tea, you can simply add a teaspoon of Maca powder to hot water, stirring well until it's fully dissolved. This tea not only boosts energy but also supports hormonal balance. Tinctures and extracts are another effective method. For a Cat's Claw tincture, the bark is soaked in alcohol for several weeks, allowing the active compounds to infuse into the liquid. This tincture can be taken in small doses to support immune health and reduce inflammation. Healing ceremonies often incorporate these plants in various forms. Shamans might use Yerba Mate in rituals to enhance mental clarity and spiritual connection, preparing it by steeping the leaves in hot water and sharing the infusion with participants.

For those interested in incorporating these remedies into their daily routine, here are some specific recipes. An energy-boosting Maca smoothie is a delicious way to start your day. Blend one teaspoon of Maca powder with a banana, a cup of almond milk, a tablespoon of peanut butter, and a drizzle of honey. This smoothie not only provides a natural energy boost but also supplies essential nutrients to support overall health. An immune-supporting Cat's Claw tincture can be made by soaking one cup of Cat's Claw bark in two cups of vodka or brandy for four to six weeks. Shake the jar daily to ensure proper infusion. After the soaking period, strain the liquid into a dark glass bottle. Take one to two teaspoons of this tincture daily to boost your immune system.

Yerba Mate infusion for mental alertness is a simple yet effective way to enhance focus and clarity. To prepare, steep one tablespoon of Yerba Mate leaves in a cup of hot water for about five minutes. Strain the leaves and enjoy the infusion. This traditional South American tea not only provides a natural caffeine boost but also delivers antioxidants that support overall health. Drink it in the morning or early afternoon to stay alert and focused throughout the day.

South American herbal healing traditions offer a rich tapestry of natural remedies deeply rooted in cultural practices. The influence of ancient civilizations, the role of shamans and traditional healers, and the integration of herbal medicine with spiritual practices have all contributed to the profound understanding of these plants' healing properties. You can benefit from their natural energy-boosting, immune-supporting, and stimulant properties by exploring and incorporating key medicinal plants like Maca, Cat's Claw, and Yerba Mate into your daily routine. The recipes provided here are a practical introduction to the powerful and time-tested remedies of South American herbal medicine.

ANCIENT EUROPEAN HERBAL LORE

As we immerse ourselves in the rich tapestry of ancient European herbalism, we uncover a tradition deeply influenced by Greek and Roman medicine. The foundations laid by Hippocrates and Galen established a systematic approach to herbal remedies, emphasizing the balance of the four humors: blood, phlegm, yellow bile, and black bile. The Greeks and Romans meticulously documented the medicinal properties of numerous plants, creating texts that served as references for centuries. This knowledge was preserved and expanded upon by monasteries during the Middle Ages. Monks and nuns meticulously transcribed ancient texts, cultivated medicinal gardens, and provided care for the sick. These monastic centers became beacons of herbal knowledge, ensuring the continuity of these practices through turbulent times.

Folk traditions and witchcraft also played a significant role in the development of European herbalism. In rural communities, wise women and cunning men used plants to heal, drawing on centuries of oral tradition. These healers often faced persecution, particularly during the witch hunts of the early modern period, yet their knowledge endured and passed down through generations. This blending of classical, monastic, and folk traditions created a rich and diverse tapestry of herbal medicine in Europe.

Among the most revered plants in ancient European herbal medicine is lavender. It's known for its soothing aroma; lavender has long been used to promote relaxation and sleep. The calming effects of lavender were well-documented in ancient texts, and it was often used in baths, sachets, and pillows to help ease the mind and encourage restful sleep. St. John's Wort, another highly valued herb, was traditionally used for mood support. This bright yellow flower, often found in meadows and along roadsides, contains compounds that affect neurotransmitters in the brain, helping to alleviate symptoms of depression and anxiety. Valerian, with its distinctive musky scent, was widely used to treat anxiety and sleep disorders. The roots of the Valerian plant contain compounds that have a sedative effect, making it a popular remedy for insomnia and nervous tension.

Traditional preparation methods for these plants were designed to extract their healing properties effectively. Herbal teas and infusions were a common way to consume these herbs. To make a relaxing lavender tea, simply steep one to two teaspoons of dried lavender flowers in a cup of hot water for about 10 minutes. This fragrant tea can be enjoyed in the evening to help unwind and prepare for sleep. Herbal baths and compresses were also widely used. A lavender bath can be made by adding a handful of dried lavender flowers to a muslin bag and placing it in the bathwater. The warm water helps to release the essential oils, creating a soothing and aromatic experience that calms the mind and relaxes the body.

Creating tinctures and extracts was another key method. For a mood-supporting St. John's Wort tincture, the flowers and buds of the plant were soaked in alcohol for several weeks, allowing the active compounds to infuse into the liquid. This tincture can be taken in small doses to help lift the mood and reduce anxiety. To prepare a sleep-enhancing Valerian infusion, add one teaspoon of dried Valerian root to a cup of hot water and let it steep for about 15 minutes. Strain the liquid and drink it about an hour before bedtime to promote restful sleep.

For those looking to explore these remedies, here are some specific recipes. Relaxing lavender tea is simple to prepare. Steep one to two teaspoons of dried lavender flowers in a cup of hot water for 10 minutes. Strain and enjoy this fragrant tea in the evening to help unwind and prepare for sleep. To make a mood-supporting St. John's Wort tincture, fill a jar with fresh St. John's Wort flowers and buds, then cover with vodka or brandy. Seal the jar and store it in a cool, dark place for four to six weeks, shaking it daily. Strain the liquid into a dark glass bottle and take one to two teaspoons daily to help lift your mood.

A sleep-enhancing Valerian infusion can be made by steeping one teaspoon of dried Valerian root in a cup of hot water for 15 minutes. Strain and drink this infusion about an hour before bedtime to promote restful sleep. The sedative properties of Valerian help to ease anxiety and prepare the mind and body for a good night's rest.

Ancient European herbal lore provides a wealth of knowledge and practices that continue to offer natural and effective solutions for modern health challenges. The influence of Greek and Roman medicine, the preservation efforts of monasteries, and the rich traditions of folk healers have all contributed to a vibrant and enduring herbal tradition. By exploring key medicinal plants like lavender, St. John's Wort, and Valerian, and understanding their traditional preparation methods, you can incorporate these time-tested remedies into your daily life. These practices not only provide natural solutions for relaxation, mood support, and sleep disorders but also connect us to the rich heritage of European herbal medicine.

As we move forward, we will delve into the practical applications of these ancient remedies, exploring how they can be seamlessly integrated into modern wellness routines.

CHAPTER 5: PRACTICAL APPLICATIONS OF HERBS

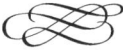

The first time I experienced the profound relaxation of an herbal bath was during a particularly stressful period in my life. I had been juggling multiple responsibilities, and my mind was constantly racing. One evening, a friend suggested I try an herbal bath to unwind. Skeptical but desperate for relief, I gathered some lavender and chamomile from my garden, prepared a simple infusion, and poured it into my bath. As I sank into the warm, fragrant water, I felt an immediate sense of calm wash over me. This experience ignited my passion for herbal baths and their myriad benefits.

HERBAL BATHS AND THEIR BENEFITS

Herbal baths have been cherished for centuries across various cultures for their therapeutic effects on the body and mind. They offer a sanctuary of relaxation and stress relief, providing a quiet escape from the pressures of daily life. Soaking in a warm bath infused with calming herbs like lavender can induce a state of tranquility, helping to alleviate anxiety and promote better sleep.

The warm water, combined with the soothing properties of herbs, creates a perfect environment for unwinding and resetting your mental state.

Beyond relaxation, herbal baths are excellent for skin health and hydration. The warm water opens your pores, allowing the beneficial compounds in the herbs to penetrate deeply. Chamomile, for example, is renowned for its ability to soothe irritated skin and reduce inflammation. It's particularly effective for conditions like eczema and dermatitis. Herbal baths also support detoxification and improve circulation. The heat from the water stimulates blood flow, helping to flush out toxins from your body. Adding herbs like rosemary can enhance this effect, as it is known to boost circulation and provide a gentle detoxifying effect.

Herbal baths can also provide relief from muscle aches and pains. The heat of the bathwater, combined with muscle-relaxing herbs like eucalyptus and rosemary, can ease tension and reduce soreness. Epsom salts, often added to herbal baths, are rich in magnesium, which helps to relax muscles and reduce inflammation. This makes herbal baths a perfect remedy for athletes or anyone suffering from chronic muscle pain.

When it comes to preparing herbal baths, there are several methods to choose from. One simple way is to make herbal infusions for your bathwater. To do this, steep your chosen herbs in boiling water for about 20 minutes, then strain the liquid and add it to your bath. This method ensures that the beneficial compounds are fully extracted and ready to be absorbed by your skin. Creating herbal bath sachets is another easy and mess-free option. Fill a small muslin bag with dried herbs, tie it securely, and place it in your bathwater. As the water heats up, the herbs will release their therapeutic properties without leaving a mess in your tub.

Adding essential oils to your bath can enhance the therapeutic effects. Essential oils are concentrated extracts from plants, and just a few drops can provide significant benefits. However, always dilute essential oils in a carrier oil or liquid Castile soap before adding them to your bath to avoid skin irritation. Tips for optimal soaking time and temperature are also crucial. The recommended water temperature for a therapeutic soak is between 100.4-105.8°F. Soak for about 20-30 minutes to allow your body to absorb the herbal benefits fully.

A relaxation bath with lavender and chamomile is perfect for unwinding after a long day. To prepare, steep one cup of dried lavender flowers and one cup of dried chamomile flowers in boiling water for 20 minutes. Strain the infusion and add it to your bathwater. This combination will help calm your mind and soothe your senses, promoting a restful night's sleep.

For a detox bath with rosemary and Epsom salts, combine two cups of Epsom salts with half a cup of dried rosemary leaves. Dissolve the mixture in your bathwater. The Epsom salts will help draw out toxins, while the rosemary boosts circulation and supports detoxification.

A respiratory relief bath with eucalyptus and peppermint is excellent for clearing nasal passages and easing congestion. Add a few drops of eucalyptus essential oil and peppermint essential oil to a carrier oil, then pour the mixture into your bath. The steam from the hot water will carry the essential oils, helping to open your airways and relieve respiratory discomfort.

For skin-soothing benefits, try a bath with oatmeal and calendula. Grind one cup of oatmeal into a fine powder and combine it with half a cup of dried calendula flowers. Place the mixture in a muslin bag and add it to your bathwater. The oatmeal will moisturize and protect your skin, while calendula helps to reduce inflammation and promote healing.

Herbal baths offer a simple yet profoundly effective way to incorporate the healing power of herbs into your daily routine. Whether you seek relaxation, detoxification, muscle relief, or skin health, there is an herbal bath recipe to meet your needs. Embrace this ancient practice and experience the therapeutic benefits for yourself.

MAKING HERBAL SYRUPS FOR COUGH AND COLD

When the chill of winter sets in and the sniffles start, one of the most comforting remedies you can turn to is herbal syrup. Herbal syrups are not just a sweet treat; they are a potent way to soothe throat irritation, ease coughs and congestion, and provide immune support. Their thick, viscous texture coats the throat, providing immediate relief from dryness and irritation. Unlike many over-the-counter medications, herbal syrups are made from natural ingredients and can be tailored to suit your specific needs.

One of the most appealing aspects of herbal syrups is their pleasant taste, making them easy to administer, especially to children. A spoonful of elderberry syrup, for instance, is not only effective in fighting off colds but also enjoyable to take. Elderberries are packed with antiviral properties, making them a powerful ally in your fight against respiratory infections. Thyme is another excellent herb for cough relief. Its expectorant effects help to loosen mucus, making it easier to clear from your respiratory tract. Licorice root, known for its soothing properties, can calm a sore throat and reduce inflammation. Ginger, with its anti-inflammatory benefits, can help ease congestion and support overall respiratory health.

Creating herbal syrups at home is a rewarding process that allows you to control the quality and potency of the ingredients. Start by making a decoction, which is a concentrated herbal tea. Combine your chosen herbs with water in a pot and bring it to a boil. Reduce the heat and let it simmer until the liquid reduces by half. This process extracts the active compounds from the herbs, creating a potent base for your syrup. Once the decoction is ready, strain out the herbs and return the liquid to the pot. Add honey or glycerin to sweeten and preserve the syrup. Honey not only acts as a natural preservative but also adds its own antibacterial properties to the mix. Stir until fully combined, then pour the syrup into sterilized glass bottles for storage. Keep your syrup in the refrigerator, where it can last for several weeks.

Dosage is important for both effectiveness and safety. For adults, a tablespoon of syrup every four hours can help manage symptoms. For children, reduce the dose to a teaspoon. Always consult with a healthcare provider before giving herbal remedies to young children or if you have any underlying health conditions.

To make an elderberry syrup for immune support:

1. Combine one cup of dried elderberries with four cups of water in a pot.
2. Bring to a boil, then reduce heat and simmer for 45 minutes.
3. Strain the liquid and discard the berries.
4. Return the liquid to the pot and add one cup of honey.
5. Stir until well mixed and pour into sterilized bottles. This syrup can be taken daily as a preventive measure or more frequently during illness.

For a thyme and honey syrup to relieve coughs, combine one cup of fresh thyme with two cups of water. Simmer for 30 minutes, strain, and return the liquid to the pot. Add one cup of honey and stir until dissolved. This syrup can be taken with a spoonful to help clear mucus and ease coughing.

A ginger and licorice root syrup for soothing sore throats can be made by simmering one cup of sliced ginger and one cup of dried licorice root in four cups of water for an hour. Strain the liquid, add one cup of honey, and stir until well combined. This soothing syrup will help reduce inflammation and ease throat pain.

For comprehensive cold relief, create a combination syrup using elderberries, thyme, ginger, and licorice root. Combine half a cup of each herb with four cups of water. Simmer until the liquid reduces by half, strain, and add one and a half cups of honey. This multi-herb syrup addresses a range of cold symptoms, from congestion and sore throat to overall immune support.

Herbal syrups are a wonderful, natural way to support your health during cold and flu season. With their soothing properties, pleasant taste, and immune-boosting benefits, they are a staple in any natural medicine cabinet. Whether you are preparing them for yourself, your children, or your elderly parents, these syrups offer a gentle yet effective remedy for respiratory ailments.

CRAFTING ESSENTIAL OILS AT HOME

The first time I crafted my own essential oils, I felt a deep connection to the plants I was using. There's something incredibly satisfying about creating these potent extracts yourself, knowing that they can be used in a variety of ways to enhance your well-being. Essential oils are revered for their therapeutic effects and versatile applications. Aromatherapy, for instance, uses the powerful scents of essential oils to promote emotional well-being. Inhaling the aroma of lavender can induce relaxation and help you sleep better, while peppermint can invigorate your senses and alleviate headaches.

Topically, essential oils offer numerous benefits for skin health. Tea tree oil, known for its antimicrobial properties, can be applied to skin infections and acne, providing a natural remedy that avoids harsh chemicals. Respiratory support is another significant benefit of essential oils.

Eucalyptus oil, when inhaled, can clear nasal passages and ease congestion, making it a staple during cold and flu season. Beyond personal care, essential oils can also be used in homemade cleaning products. Lemon oil, with its uplifting scent and antibacterial properties, can be added to cleaning solutions to naturally disinfect surfaces and leave your home smelling fresh.

Several herbs are particularly effective for producing essential oils. Lavender is widely celebrated for its calming effects, making it ideal for relaxation and sleep aids. Peppermint, with its cooling and refreshing properties, is excellent for relieving headaches and nausea. Tea tree oil is a versatile antimicrobial agent, effective against a wide range of bacteria and fungi. Lemon oil not only uplifts your mood but also serves as a powerful cleaning agent, making it a must-have in any natural cleaning arsenal.

The process of extracting essential oils can be both fascinating and rewarding. Steam distillation is the most common method. It involves placing plant material in a distillation apparatus, where steam is passed through. The steam helps release the volatile aromatic compounds, which then condense into liquid form. This liquid is collected in a separator, where the essential oil can be siphoned off from the water. Cold pressing is another technique that is particularly useful for citrus peels. It involves mechanically pressing the peels to release their oils. This method is simple yet effective, capturing the vibrant essence of citrus fruits.

To ensure you maximize the yield and purity of your essential oils, it's crucial to use proper equipment and follow safety precautions. Always use high-quality, stainless steel or glass apparatus to avoid contamination. Ensure that your workspace is clean and free from debris. Maintaining a consistent temperature and pressure during extraction can help optimize the quality of your oils. Additionally, store your essential oils in dark glass bottles to protect them from light and air, which can degrade their potency over time.

A popular recipe for lavender oil involves using the steam distillation method. Gather fresh or dried lavender flowers and place them in the distillation apparatus. Pass steam through the plant material, allowing the steam to capture the aromatic compounds. As the steam condenses, the liquid is collected in a separator. Once the essential oil separates from the water, siphon it into a dark glass bottle for storage. This lavender oil can be used as a sleep aid by adding a few drops to your pillow or diffusing it in your bedroom.

Peppermint oil can be crafted through cold pressing. Collect fresh peppermint leaves and press them mechanically to extract the oil. This invigorating oil is perfect for relieving headaches. Simply dilute a few drops in a carrier oil and massage it onto your temples for quick relief. Tea tree oil, known for its antimicrobial properties, can be made using steam distillation. The oil is highly effective for treating skin infections and acne. Dilute it with a carrier oil and apply it to the affected area for natural healing.

Lemon oil, with its refreshing scent and cleaning power, can be extracted using cold pressing. Collect the peels of fresh lemons and press them to release the oil. This oil can be added to homemade cleaning solutions to disinfect surfaces and uplift your mood. Mix a few drops with water and vinegar for an effective and natural cleaning spray.

Crafting your own essential oils at home allows you to harness the powerful benefits of these natural extracts. Whether you use them for aromatherapy, skin care, respiratory support, or cleaning, essential oils offer a versatile and effective way to incorporate the healing properties of herbs into your daily life.

HOMEMADE HERBAL LOTIONS AND CREAMS

Herbal lotions and creams offer a natural way to care for your skin, providing hydration, healing, and protection against environmental damage. Unlike commercial products that often contain synthetic chemicals and preservatives, homemade herbal lotions are made from natural ingredients that nourish your skin. They are particularly beneficial for those seeking a chemical-free skincare routine. One of the primary benefits of herbal lotions is their ability to hydrate and moisturize the skin. Ingredients like almond oil and coconut oil penetrate deeply, providing lasting moisture without clogging pores. This hydration is essential for maintaining the skin's elasticity and preventing dryness and flakiness.

Herbal lotions and creams also possess healing and soothing properties.

Herbs like calendula and chamomile are known for their anti-inflammatory and wound-healing effects. Calendula, often used in salves and creams, helps to soothe irritated skin and promote the healing of minor cuts and abrasions. Chamomile, with its gentle anti-inflammatory properties, is perfect for sensitive skin, reducing redness and calming irritation. Aloe vera is another key ingredient, renowned for its cooling and hydrating effects. It is particularly effective in treating sunburns, providing immediate relief, and promoting faster healing.

Moreover, herbal lotions offer protection against environmental damage. Rosemary, with its antioxidant properties, helps to combat the effects of free radicals, which can accelerate the aging process. Regular use of rosemary-infused lotions can help to maintain youthful skin and protect it from the harmful effects of pollution and UV radiation. These natural formulations provide a barrier that shields the skin while allowing it to breathe, unlike many commercial products that can suffocate the skin with synthetic compounds.

To make your own herbal lotions and creams, start by infusing oils with medicinal herbs. This process involves soaking dried herbs in a carrier oil, such as olive or almond oil, for several weeks. The oil absorbs the beneficial compounds from the herbs, resulting in a potent, herbal-infused oil. Heat the oil gently in a double boiler to speed up the infusion process, then strain out the herbs. Next, combine the infused oil with beeswax and emulsifiers to create a stable lotion. Beeswax not only thickens the lotion but also adds protective and moisturizing properties. Melt the beeswax in a double boiler, then slowly add the infused oil, stirring constantly to combine.

Adding essential oils enhances the benefits of your lotion. Essential oils like lavender, tea tree, and frankincense can provide additional healing, soothing, and anti-aging properties. Always dilute essential oils properly to avoid skin irritation. Once your lotion is well mixed, pour it into sterilized glass jars or bottles for storage. Store your herbal lotions in a cool, dark place to prolong their shelf life.

For a healing calendula lotion designed for dry skin, infuse one cup of dried calendula flowers in one cup of olive oil. Strain the oil after two weeks. Melt one ounce of beeswax in a double boiler, then slowly add the calendula-infused oil, stirring until well combined. Add a few drops of lavender essential oil for added soothing effects. Pour the mixture into jars and let it cool completely before using. This lotion will provide deep hydration and help to heal dry, cracked skin.

A soothing chamomile cream for sensitive skin can be made by infusing one cup of dried chamomile flowers in one cup of almond oil. After straining, melt half an ounce of beeswax and combine it with the chamomile-infused oil. Stir in a few drops of chamomile essential oil to enhance the calming properties. This cream will reduce redness and irritation, making it perfect for those with sensitive or reactive skin.

For sunburn relief, a hydrating aloe vera gel is ideal. Start with one cup of fresh aloe vera gel and blend until smooth. In a double boiler, melt half an ounce of beeswax and add one cup of coconut oil. Once combined, remove from heat and stir in the aloe vera gel. Add a few drops of peppermint essential oil for a cooling effect. This gel will soothe sunburned skin and provide much-needed hydration.

An anti-aging rosemary and green tea cream can be crafted by infusing one cup of dried rosemary leaves in one cup of grapeseed oil. Strain the oil and melt one ounce of beeswax in a double boiler. Combine the rosemary-infused oil with half a cup of strong green tea. Stir in a few drops of frankincense essential oil. This cream will help combat the signs of aging, providing antioxidant protection and promoting youthful, radiant skin.

CAPSULES AND TABLETS: MODERN TAKES ON ANCIENT REMEDIES

Herbal capsules and tablets offer a modern, convenient way to incorporate the benefits of ancient remedies into your daily routine. One of the primary advantages of these forms is their easy dosage and portability. Unlike liquid extracts or teas, capsules can be taken on the go, fitting seamlessly into a busy lifestyle. They also provide a long shelf life and stability, ensuring that the active compounds remain potent over time. This makes them an ideal choice for those who want to maintain a consistent herbal regimen without worrying about spoilage.

The targeted delivery of active compounds is another significant benefit. Capsules and tablets allow for precise dosing, ensuring that you receive the exact amount of the herb needed for therapeutic effects. This is particularly useful for herbs that require specific dosages to be effective. Additionally, capsules and tablets minimize taste and odor issues, which can be a concern with some herbal preparations. For instance, while turmeric is highly beneficial for its anti-inflammatory properties, its strong taste can be off-putting for some. Encapsulating it removes this barrier, making it easier to consume regularly.

Several herbs are particularly suited for encapsulation due to their potent properties. Turmeric is a prime example, renowned for its anti-inflammatory effects. It contains curcumin, a compound that has been extensively studied for its ability to reduce inflammation and provide pain relief. Ashwagandha, another popular herb, is known for its ability to combat stress and enhance vitality. It works as an adaptogen, helping the body to cope with physical and mental stressors. Milk thistle is widely used for liver support, aiding in detoxification and protecting liver cells from damage. Valerian is an excellent herb for those struggling with sleep and anxiety, promoting relaxation and improving sleep quality.

Making herbal capsules and tablets at home is a straightforward process that allows you to control the quality and dosage of the herbs. Start by grinding the herbs into a fine powder using a coffee grinder or mortar and pestle. This ensures that the active compounds are evenly distributed throughout the capsule. Next, select the appropriate capsule size and type. Vegetarian or gelatin capsules are commonly available and can be chosen based on personal preference. Using a capsule-filling machine can greatly simplify the process, allowing you to fill multiple capsules at once and ensure consistent dosage.

To make anti-inflammatory turmeric capsules, begin by grinding dried turmeric root into a fine powder. Fill the capsules using a capsule-filling machine, ensuring each capsule contains about 500 milligrams of turmeric powder. For added benefits, you can mix in a small amount of black pepper, which enhances the absorption of curcumin in the body. Store the filled capsules in a dark, cool place to maintain their potency.

Stress-relief ashwagandha tablets can be made by grinding dried ashwagandha root into a fine powder. Combine the powder with a binding agent, such as acacia gum or honey, to form a dough-like consistency. Press the mixture into tablet molds and allow them to dry completely. These tablets can be taken daily to help manage stress and improve overall vitality.

For liver support, milk thistle capsules are an excellent choice. Grind dried milk thistle seeds into a fine powder and fill the capsules using a capsule-filling machine. Each capsule should contain about 250 milligrams of milk thistle powder. These capsules can be taken daily to support liver health and detoxification.

Sleep aid valerian root tablets can be made by grinding dried valerian root into a fine powder. Mix the powder with a small amount of honey or another binding agent to form a dough. Press the mixture into tablet molds and allow them to dry. Taking one of these tablets before bed can help promote relaxation and improve sleep quality.

Herbal capsules and tablets offer a convenient and effective way to integrate the healing power of herbs into your daily routine. Whether you are seeking anti-inflammatory benefits, stress relief, liver support, or better sleep, these forms provide a practical solution for consistent and targeted herbal therapy.

PREPARING HERBAL RUBS FOR PAIN RELIEF

Herbal rubs stand out as a natural solution for pain relief and muscle recovery. By applying them directly to the skin, you can target specific areas of discomfort. This method allows the active compounds in the herbs to penetrate through the skin, delivering their therapeutic effects right where they are needed most. Unlike synthetic painkillers, herbal rubs offer a soothing and warming sensation, providing relief without side effects. The warmth helps relax muscles, while the herbs reduce inflammation and pain. This makes herbal rubs a perfect choice for those seeking a natural and chemical-free approach to pain management.

Several herbs are particularly effective for making herbal rubs. Arnica is well-known for its ability to reduce bruising and inflammation. It has been used for centuries to treat sprains, strains, and other injuries. Cayenne, with its active compound capsaicin, provides a warming effect that helps to alleviate pain. It is especially useful for chronic conditions like arthritis and muscle pain. Comfrey is another valuable herb known for promoting healing and tissue repair. It contains allantoin, which stimulates cell growth and helps to mend broken bones and torn tissues. Peppermint, with its cooling and soothing effects, is excellent for relieving sore muscles and tension headaches.

To make herbal rubs, start by infusing oils with your chosen medicinal herbs. This process involves placing dried herbs in a jar and covering them with a carrier oil, such as olive or coconut oil. Seal the jar and let it sit in a warm, sunny spot for several weeks, shaking it daily to encourage the infusion. Once the oil is ready, strain out the herbs and combine the infused oil with beeswax or other thickeners to achieve the desired consistency. Beeswax thickens the rub and adds a protective layer to the skin. Adding essential oils can enhance the benefits of your rub. For instance, lavender essential oil can provide additional pain relief and relaxation.

Proper storage and application techniques are crucial for maintaining the effectiveness of your herbal rubs. Store them in airtight containers, preferably dark glass jars, to protect them from light and air. Keep them in a cool, dark place to prolong their shelf life. When applying the rub, gently and circularly massage it into the affected area. This helps the skin absorb the beneficial compounds and promotes blood circulation, enhancing the overall effect.

For an arnica and cayenne muscle rub, start by infusing one cup of dried arnica flowers in one cup of olive oil. After straining, heat the infused oil with one tablespoon of cayenne powder in a double boiler for about 30 minutes. Strain the mixture again to remove any remaining particles. Melt one ounce of beeswax in the double boiler, then slowly add the infused oil, stirring until well combined. Add a few drops of peppermint essential oil for a cooling effect. Pour the mixture into jars and let it cool completely before using. This rub is perfect for relieving muscle pain and inflammation.

A comfrey and peppermint joint relief balm can be made by infusing one cup of dried comfrey leaves in one cup of coconut oil. Strain the oil after two weeks. In a double boiler, melt half an ounce of beeswax and combine it with the comfrey-infused oil. Add a few drops of peppermint essential oil for its cooling and soothing properties. This balm is excellent for joint pain and can be applied directly to the affected area for relief.

For a warming ginger and turmeric pain-relief salve, start by infusing one cup of dried ginger root and one cup of dried turmeric root in one cup of almond oil. Strain the oil and heat it in a double boiler with one ounce of beeswax. Once combined, add a few drops of clove essential oil for its additional warming effects. This salve is ideal for chronic pain conditions, providing both warmth and anti-inflammatory benefits.

A cooling menthol and eucalyptus rub for sore muscles can be crafted by infusing one cup of dried eucalyptus leaves in one cup of grapeseed oil. Strain the oil and melt half an ounce of beeswax in a double boiler. Combine the infused oil with the beeswax and add a few drops of menthol essential oil. This rub provides a cooling sensation that helps to relieve muscle soreness and tension.

In the next chapter, we will explore the principles of preventative health and immunity, delving into how herbs can support long-term well-being and resilience.

CHAPTER 6: PREVENTATIVE HEALTH AND IMMUNITY

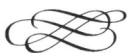

Several years ago, during a particularly harsh winter, I found myself battling one cold after another. Frustrated with the constant cycle of illness, I reached out to a friend who was well-versed in herbal medicine. She introduced me to the concept of daily tonics—simple, nourishing herbal concoctions designed to bolster the immune system and enhance overall vitality. I incorporated these tonics into my daily routine, and the difference was remarkable. That winter was the last time I faced such frequent illnesses. This chapter delves into the powerful world of daily tonics and how they can become a cornerstone of your health regimen.

DAILY TONICS FOR IMMUNE SUPPORT

Daily tonics are more than just herbal teas; they are potent, carefully crafted blends that you consume regularly to support your immune system and overall health. The key to their effectiveness lies in consistency. Unlike occasional herbal teas, which you might drink sporadically, daily tonics are meant to be a staple in your routine. Consistent intake allows your body to build up its defenses over time, leading to long-term benefits. These tonics work by nourishing your body with essential vitamins, minerals, and bioactive compounds that promote resilience and vitality.

Historically, cultures around the world have used daily tonics as a preventative measure against illness. In traditional Chinese medicine, tonic herbs like astragalus are consumed regularly to strengthen the body's defenses. Similarly, in Ayurvedic practices, daily tonics made from herbs like ashwagandha are used to maintain balance and vitality. These traditions recognize that ongoing, daily support is crucial for maintaining health and preventing disease.

Several herbs stand out for their immune-boosting properties and are particularly effective when used in daily tonics. Astragalus is a powerhouse herb known for its ability to enhance immune function. Studies have shown that it can increase the production of white blood cells, which are crucial for fighting off infections. Elderberry is another excellent choice, revered for its antiviral properties. It has been used traditionally to reduce the severity and duration of colds and flu. Echinacea is well-known for stimulating the immune response, making it a popular choice during cold and flu season. Reishi mushroom, often called the "mushroom of immortality," supports overall immunity and has adaptogenic properties that help the body cope with stress.

To incorporate these herbs into your daily routine, you can prepare them as decoctions or infusions. A decoction involves simmering the herbs in water to extract their active compounds. This method is particularly effective for tough, fibrous plant materials like roots and mushrooms. For instance, to make an astragalus and reishi immune tonic, combine dried astragalus root and reishi mushroom slices with water, bring to a boil, then simmer for about 30 minutes. Strain the liquid and drink it daily. Infusions, on the other hand, are made by steeping the herbs in hot water, which is ideal for more delicate plant parts like flowers and leaves.

When preparing daily tonics, you can experiment with both hot and cold preparations. For a cold infusion, place the herbs in cold water and let them steep overnight in the refrigerator. This method is particularly refreshing in warmer months and preserves some of the more volatile compounds that might be lost in hot water. Combining herbs can also enhance their synergistic effects. For example, an elderberry and ginger daily health tonic combines the antiviral properties of elderberry with the warming, anti-inflammatory benefits of ginger.

Proper storage and dosage are essential for maintaining the potency and effectiveness of your daily tonics. Store your prepared tonics in airtight glass containers in the refrigerator, where they can last for several days. For dried herbs, keep them in a cool, dark place to preserve their medicinal properties. As for dosage, a general recommendation is to drink one to two cups of tonic daily, but you can adjust based on your body's needs and response.

Here are some specific recipes to get you started. For an astragalus and reishi immune tonic, combine one tablespoon of dried astragalus root and one tablespoon of reishi mushroom slices with four cups of water. Simmer for 30 minutes, strain, and drink one cup daily. For an elderberry and ginger daily health tonic, simmer one cup of dried elderberries and a two-inch piece of fresh ginger in four cups of water for 20 minutes. Strain and enjoy a cup each day. An echinacea and lemon balm infusion can be made by steeping one tablespoon of dried echinacea and one tablespoon of dried lemon balm in hot water for 15 minutes. Drink this infusion once or twice daily. Finally, a multi-herb immune-boosting tonic can be created by combining equal parts of astragalus, elderberry, echinacea, and reishi. Simmer one tablespoon of this blend in four cups of water for 30 minutes, strain, and drink one cup daily.

Incorporating these daily tonics into your routine can profoundly impact your health. By providing consistent, nourishing support to your immune system, you can enhance your body's natural defenses and enjoy greater vitality and resilience.

SEASONAL HERBS FOR COLD AND FLU PREVENTION

As the seasons change, so do our bodies' needs. The shift from winter's chill to spring's bloom, summer's heat, and autumn's cool can impact our immune health in significant ways. Seasonal herbs can play a crucial role in keeping colds and flu at bay, tailored to the specific demands of each time of year. Spring, for instance, brings allergies and a need for detoxification after winter, while summer focuses on cooling and respiratory health. Fall is the time to bolster immunity for the coming cold months, and winter requires warming and circulation-boosting herbs. Traditional medicine has long advocated for seasonal eating and herbal use, recognizing the body's different requirements throughout the year. This proactive, seasonal approach to herbal support can enhance your health and prevent common illnesses.

In spring, elderflower emerges as an effective herb for combating allergies and boosting immunity. It's known for its anti-inflammatory properties; elderflower can alleviate hay fever symptoms and other seasonal allergies. Preparing an immune-boosting tea with elderflower and nettle can help clear toxins accumulated over winter and strengthen your body's defenses. Simply steep one tablespoon each of dried elderflower and nettle in hot water for 10-15 minutes. Drink this infusion daily to support your body during the spring months.

As autumn arrives, echinacea becomes a valuable ally in preparing your immune system for the colder weather. This herb is renowned for stimulating the immune response, making it a go-to remedy during the fall. To make an echinacea and elderberry syrup:

1. Combine one cup of dried echinacea root and one cup of dried elderberries with four cups of water.
2. Simmer for 30 minutes, strain, and add honey to taste.
3. Store the syrup in the refrigerator and take one tablespoon daily to fortify your immune system against the impending flu season.

Winter calls for warming herbs that boost circulation and provide comfort against the cold.

Ginger is particularly effective in this regard, offering both anti-inflammatory and circulatory benefits. A warming ginger and cinnamon tea can be a delightful way to stave off winter chills. Simply slice a two-inch piece of fresh ginger and add it to two cups of water. Bring to a boil, add a cinnamon stick, and simmer for 10 minutes. Strain and enjoy a cup of this spicy, warming tea daily to keep your body warm and your immune system strong.

Summer, with its heat and potential for respiratory issues, benefits from cooling and soothing herbs. Peppermint, known for its refreshing properties, can help clear nasal passages and cool the body. A summer-cooling peppermint and lemon balm infusion is refreshing and effective. Steep one tablespoon of dried peppermint and one tablespoon of dried lemon balm in hot water for 10-15 minutes. This infusion can be enjoyed hot or cold, providing relief from the summer heat and supporting respiratory health.

Incorporating these seasonal herbs into your routine involves various preparation methods. Herbal teas and infusions are simple yet effective ways to consume these herbs. For a seasonal tea, steep the herbs in hot water, cover them and let them infuse for the recommended time. Herbal syrups and tinctures offer a more concentrated form of these herbs. To make a syrup, simmer the herbs in water, strain, and add honey or glycerin. Tinctures involve soaking herbs in alcohol for several weeks, then straining and bottling the liquid.

Creating herbal steams and inhalations can provide immediate relief for respiratory issues. For a steam, add a few drops of essential oil or a handful of dried herbs to a bowl of hot water. Lean over the bowl, cover your head with a towel, and inhale the steam. This method is particularly effective with eucalyptus or peppermint for clearing nasal congestion.

Combining herbs based on seasonal needs can enhance their effectiveness. For example, a spring tea might combine elderflower, nettle, and dandelion for a comprehensive detox and allergy relief. A fall syrup could mix echinacea, elderberry, and ginger for robust immune support. By tailoring your herbal remedies to the seasons, you can provide your body with the specific support it needs throughout the year.

HERBAL REMEDIES FOR BOOSTING ENERGY

Herbs play a significant role in boosting both physical and mental energy, offering a natural alternative to synthetic stimulants. Unlike caffeine or sugar, which provide a quick but short-lived spike in energy, certain herbs work with your body's systems to enhance endurance and vitality over the long term. Adaptogens are a unique class of herbs that help the body adapt to stress, balancing cortisol levels and supporting adrenal health. This balancing act reduces fatigue and promotes sustained energy without the crash that often follows conventional stimulants. Over time, these herbs can improve overall resilience, making you feel more energized and focused throughout the day.

Ginseng is one of the most renowned herbs for boosting vitality and endurance. Its adaptogenic properties help improve stamina and reduce fatigue by enhancing the body's ability to handle stress. Rhodiola, another powerful adaptogen, is known for its ability to reduce fatigue and improve mental focus. It has been used for centuries in traditional medicine to combat the physical and mental toll of stress. Maca, a root native to the Andes, is celebrated for its ability to balance hormones and provide a natural energy boost. It is particularly effective for those experiencing hormonal imbalances that contribute to fatigue. Ashwagandha is another excellent herb for stress reduction and sustained energy, helping to lower cortisol levels and support overall adrenal function.

Preparing and using these herbs for energy support can be both simple and versatile. Herbal teas and decoctions are a straightforward way to incorporate these herbs into your daily routine. To make a ginseng and Rhodiola energy tonic, combine dried ginseng root and Rhodiola in a pot with water, bring to a boil, and then simmer for about 20 minutes. Strain and drink a cup daily for a steady energy boost. Tinctures and extracts are another convenient option, offering a more concentrated form of these herbs. To prepare a Maca and Ashwagandha tincture, soak the powdered herbs in alcohol for several weeks, then strain and store in a dark glass bottle. A few drops added to your morning smoothie can provide a lasting energy lift.

Herbal smoothies and tonics offer a delicious and nutritious way to enjoy the benefits of these energy-boosting herbs. For a Maca and cacao smoothie, blend a teaspoon of Maca powder with a tablespoon of cacao, a banana, and a cup of almond milk. This combination boosts energy and provides a rich source of antioxidants. Another favorite is the Ashwagandha and turmeric golden milk, which combines turmeric's anti-inflammatory benefits with Ashwagandha's stress-reducing properties. Simply mix a teaspoon of each herb with warm milk and honey for a comforting and energizing drink.

Combining herbs can maximize their energy-boosting effects. Ginseng, green tea, and peppermint make a synergistic tea blend that enhances physical and mental energy. To prepare, steep a teaspoon of each herb in hot water for about 10 minutes. This blend boosts energy and provides a refreshing and invigorating flavor.

Here are some specific recipes to get you started. For a ginseng and Rhodiola energy tonic, combine a tablespoon of dried ginseng root and a tablespoon of dried Rhodiola with four cups of water. Simmer for 20 minutes, strain, and drink a cup daily. For a Maca and cacao smoothie, blend a teaspoon of Maca powder, a tablespoon of cacao, one banana, and a cup of almond milk until smooth. For Ashwagandha and turmeric golden milk, mix a teaspoon of Ashwagandha powder and a teaspoon of turmeric powder with warm milk and a spoonful of honey. Finally, for a herbal tea blend, steep a teaspoon each of ginseng, green tea, and peppermint in hot water for 10 minutes.

Incorporating these herbal remedies into your routine can provide a natural, sustainable boost to your energy levels, helping you feel more vibrant and focused every day.

NATURAL DETOXIFICATION WITH HERBS

Detoxification is a crucial process for maintaining overall health and well-being. Our bodies are exposed to a variety of toxins daily, from pollutants in the air to chemicals in our food and water. Over time, these toxins can accumulate and strain our internal systems, particularly the liver and kidneys, which are responsible for filtering and removing these harmful substances. Regular detoxification helps to remove these toxins, supporting the liver and kidneys in their vital functions. Additionally, detoxification promotes better skin health by clearing out impurities and can improve digestion by reducing the burden on the digestive system.

Various cultures have long recognized the importance of detoxification. Traditional Chinese Medicine, for instance, incorporates detoxifying herbs in seasonal cleanses to align with the body's natural rhythms. Similarly, Ayurvedic practices include detoxifying treatments like Panchakarma to purify the body and mind. These time-honored practices underscore the significance of regular detoxification for maintaining health and preventing disease.

Several herbs are particularly effective in supporting natural detoxification. Dandelion root is renowned for its ability to cleanse the liver and kidneys. It acts as a diuretic, helping to flush out toxins through urine. Milk Thistle is another powerful herb for liver protection and regeneration. It contains silymarin, a compound known for its antioxidant and anti-inflammatory properties, which helps to repair and regenerate liver cells. Burdock root is excellent for blood purification. It helps to eliminate toxins from the bloodstream and supports overall skin health. Cilantro is particularly useful for heavy metal detoxification. It binds to heavy metals like mercury and lead, facilitating their elimination from the body.

Preparing and using these detoxifying herbs can be simple and versatile. Herbal teas and decoctions are an effective way to consume these herbs. To make a liver-supporting dandelion root tea, steep one tablespoon of dried dandelion root in hot water for 10-15 minutes. Drink this tea daily to support liver and kidney function. Herbal smoothies and juices offer another delicious way to incorporate detoxifying herbs. For a Milk Thistle detox smoothie, blend a teaspoon of Milk Thistle powder with a cup of spinach, half a banana, and a cup of almond milk. This smoothie not only supports liver health but also provides essential nutrients.

Creating detox baths and topical applications can enhance the detoxification process. A detox bath with Epsom salts and baking soda can help to draw out toxins through the skin. Simply add a cup of Epsom salts and half a cup of baking soda to your bathwater and soak for 20-30 minutes. Adding a few drops of essential oils like lavender or eucalyptus can further enhance the experience.

Combining herbs for comprehensive detox support can amplify their effects. For example, a Burdock root and red clover blood-purifying tea combines the detoxifying properties of Burdock root with the cleansing benefits of red clover. Simply steep one tablespoon each of Burdock root and red clover in hot water for 10-15 minutes. Drink this tea daily to support blood purification and overall detoxification.

Here are some specific detox recipes to get you started. For a liver-supporting dandelion root tea, steep one tablespoon of dried dandelion root in hot water for 10-15 minutes. Drink this tea daily to support liver and kidney function. For a Milk Thistle detox smoothie, blend a teaspoon of Milk Thistle powder with a cup of spinach, half a banana, and a cup of almond milk. This smoothie not only supports liver health but also provides essential nutrients. A Burdock root and red clover blood-purifying tea can be made by steeping one tablespoon each of Burdock root and red clover in hot water for 10-15 minutes. Drink this tea daily to support blood purification and overall detoxification. For a cilantro and parsley heavy metal detox juice, blend a handful of fresh cilantro and parsley with a cup of water and a squeeze of lemon juice. Drink this juice daily to help eliminate heavy metals from the body.

Regular detoxification with these herbs can support your body's natural processes, helping to maintain optimal health and well-being. By incorporating these simple yet effective practices into your routine, you can enhance your body's ability to handle toxins and enjoy improved vitality and resilience.

ADAPTOGENIC HERBS FOR STRESS MANAGEMENT

Adaptogens are a unique group of herbs known for their ability to help the body adapt to stress. Unlike other herbs that target specific symptoms, adaptogens work by supporting the body's overall resilience and balance. They achieve this by modulating the body's stress response and supporting adrenal health, which plays a crucial role in hormone regulation. Over time, using adaptogens can lead to long-term benefits, such as reduced anxiety, improved mood, and enhanced energy levels. Historically, various cultures have utilized adaptogens for centuries, recognizing their ability to enhance physical and mental endurance. For instance, traditional

Chinese medicine and Ayurveda have long revered adaptogens for their balancing properties.

Ashwagandha is a powerful adaptogen known for its ability to reduce anxiety and stress. It works by lowering cortisol levels, the hormone responsible for stress. Holy Basil, also known as Tulsi, promotes calm and resilience. It helps to balance cortisol levels and supports the immune system, making it a great herb for managing stress. Rhodiola is another adaptogenic herb that enhances mood and reduces fatigue. It improves mental clarity and focus, making it particularly useful for those who experience stress-related cognitive difficulties. Schisandra, often called the "five-flavor berry," is renowned for its ability to enhance overall stress resistance and energy. It supports the adrenal glands and helps the body cope with physical and emotional stress.

Incorporating adaptogenic herbs into your routine can be both simple and effective. One way to use these herbs is by preparing adaptogenic teas and infusions. For instance, an Ashwagandha and Holy Basil calming tea can be made by steeping one teaspoon of dried Ashwagandha root and one teaspoon of dried Holy Basil in hot water for 10-15 minutes. This tea can be consumed daily to promote relaxation and reduce stress. Another method is preparing tinctures and extracts, which offer a more concentrated form of the herbs. To make a Rhodiola and Schisandra stress-relief tonic, soak equal parts of dried Rhodiola root and Schisandra berries in alcohol for several weeks, then strain and store in a dark glass bottle. A few drops of this tonic can be added to water or tea for a potent stress-relief remedy.

Adaptogenic smoothies and tonics are another delicious and nutritious way to enjoy the benefits of these herbs. For an adaptogenic smoothie, blend one teaspoon of Ashwagandha powder, one teaspoon of Maca powder, a banana, and a cup of almond milk.

This smoothie not only helps to reduce stress but also provides a natural energy boost. Combining adaptogens can maximize their stress-supporting effects. For example, an herbal blend for daily stress management can include equal parts of Ashwagandha, Holy Basil, Rhodiola, and Schisandra. This blend can be used to make teas and tinctures or added to smoothies, providing comprehensive support for stress management.

Here are some specific recipes to get you started. For an Ashwagandha and Holy Basil calming tea, steep one teaspoon of dried Ashwagandha root and one teaspoon of dried Holy Basil in hot water for 10-15 minutes. Drink this tea daily to promote relaxation and reduce stress. For a Rhodiola and Schisandra stress-relief tonic, soak equal parts of dried Rhodiola root and Schisandra berries in alcohol for several weeks, then strain and store in a dark glass bottle. Add a few drops of water or tea for a potent stress-relief remedy. To make an adaptogenic smoothie, blend one teaspoon of Ashwagandha powder, one teaspoon of Maca powder, a banana, and a cup of almond milk. This smoothie not only helps to reduce stress but also provides a natural energy boost. Combine equal parts of Ashwagandha, Holy Basil, Rhodiola, and Schisandra for an herbal blend for daily stress management. Use this blend to make teas and tinctures or add to smoothies for comprehensive stress support.

HERBAL STRATEGIES FOR ANTI-AGING

As the years go by, many of us seek ways to maintain our vitality and youthful appearance. Herbs can play a significant role in this endeavor, offering natural solutions to support healthy aging and reduce the signs of aging. One of the key benefits of herbs in anti-aging is their rich antioxidant content. Antioxidants combat free radicals and unstable molecules that can damage cells and accelerate aging. By neutralizing these free radicals, antioxidants help protect our skin and other tissues from oxidative stress, a major contributor to aging.

Herbs also support skin health and elasticity, crucial factors in maintaining a youthful appearance. For instance, herbs like Gotu Kola are known for their ability to boost collagen production, which keeps the skin firm and reduces wrinkles. Additionally, certain herbs can enhance cognitive function and memory, helping to keep our minds sharp as we age. Ginkgo Biloba, for example, has been shown to improve blood flow to the brain, supporting mental clarity and memory retention. Traditional practices across various cultures have long utilized herbs for their anti-aging benefits, from the ancient Chinese use of Reishi mushroom for longevity to the Ayurvedic use of Turmeric for its anti-inflammatory properties.

Several herbs are particularly effective in supporting healthy aging. Ginkgo Biloba stands out for its ability to enhance cognitive function and memory. It improves circulation and has neuroprotective effects, making it a valuable ally in maintaining mental sharpness. Turmeric, with its powerful anti-inflammatory and antioxidant properties, helps to reduce inflammation and oxidative stress, two key factors in the aging process. Gotu Kola is renowned for its ability to support skin health and regeneration. It promotes collagen production and improves skin elasticity, helping to reduce the appearance of wrinkles. Reishi mushroom, often referred to as the "mushroom of immortality," supports overall longevity and vitality. It has adaptogenic properties that help the body cope with stress and enhance immune function.

To incorporate these anti-aging herbs into your routine, you can prepare them in various ways. Herbal teas and infusions are a simple and effective method. For instance, a Ginkgo Biloba and green tea infusion can be made by steeping a teaspoon of dried Ginkgo Biloba leaves and a teaspoon of green tea in hot water for 10-15 minutes. This infusion supports cognitive function and provides a rich source of antioxidants. Tinctures and extracts offer a more concentrated form of these herbs. To prepare a Turmeric and ginger anti-inflammatory tonic, soak equal parts of Turmeric root and fresh ginger in alcohol for several weeks, then strain and store in a dark glass bottle. A few drops of this tonic can be added to water or tea for a potent anti-inflammatory boost.

Creating herbal skincare products can also enhance your anti-aging regimen. A Gotu Kola and aloe vera skin-rejuvenating serum can be made by blending Gotu Kola extract with fresh aloe vera gel. This serum can be applied to the face daily to promote collagen production and improve skin elasticity. Additionally, Reishi mushrooms can be used to make a longevity elixir. Simmer dried Reishi mushroom slices in water for 30 minutes, strain, and drink a cup daily to support overall vitality and longevity.

Combining these herbs can amplify their anti-aging effects. For comprehensive support, you can create a blend that includes Ginkgo Biloba, Turmeric, Gotu Kola, and Reishi mushroom. This blend can be used to make teas and tinctures or added to skincare products, providing a holistic approach to healthy aging.

Here are some specific recipes to get you started. For a Ginkgo Biloba and green tea memory support infusion, steep a teaspoon of dried Ginkgo Biloba leaves and a teaspoon of green tea in hot water for 10-15 minutes. Drink this infusion daily to support cognitive function and memory. For a Turmeric and ginger anti-inflammatory tonic, soak equal parts of Turmeric root and fresh ginger in alcohol for several weeks, then strain and store in a dark glass bottle. Add a few drops of water or tea for a potent anti-inflammatory boost. To make a Gotu Kola and aloe vera skin-rejuvenating serum, blend Gotu Kola extract with fresh aloe vera gel and apply to the face

daily. Finally, for a Reishi mushroom longevity elixir, simmer dried Reishi mushroom slices in water for 30 minutes, strain, and drink a cup daily to support overall vitality and longevity.

Incorporating these herbal strategies into your daily routine can help you maintain your vitality and youthful appearance. By leveraging the natural power of these herbs, you can support healthy aging from the inside out.

CHAPTER 7: SAFETY AND SUSTAINABILITY IN HERBAL MEDICINE

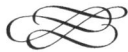

The first time I visited a bustling herbal market, I was struck by the vibrant colors and intoxicating scents of the herbs on display. Each vendor seemed to vie for attention, extolling the virtues of their wares with enthusiasm. As I wandered through the aisles, I realized that the quality of these herbs varied widely. This experience opened my eyes to the importance of sourcing high-quality herbs for effective and safe herbal medicine. In this chapter, we'll explore how to identify and source the best herbs, ensuring that your herbal remedies are both potent and safe.

IDENTIFYING AND SOURCING QUALITY HERBS

The quality of herbs you use in your remedies is paramount. High-quality herbs ensure that your preparations are effective and safe. The potency of an herb can significantly impact its therapeutic benefits. Fresh and properly harvested herbs retain active compounds, which are crucial for their medicinal properties. For instance, a fresh peppermint leaf will have a much stronger aroma and flavor compared to a dried, old one. This potency translates directly to the effectiveness of the remedy you are preparing.

Moreover, using high-quality herbs helps you avoid contaminants and adulterants. If herbs are not sourced and processed correctly, they can be contaminated with pesticides, heavy metals, or even other plant species. These contaminants not only reduce the efficacy of the herbs but can also pose serious health risks. Ensuring that your herbs are free from such contaminants is crucial for the safety of your remedies.

Another critical factor is consistency in herbal preparations. High-quality herbs provide consistent levels of active compounds, ensuring that each batch of your remedy is as effective as the last. This consistency is vital, especially when preparing remedies for specific health conditions. If the potency of your herbs varies, so will the effectiveness of your remedies.

Supporting ethical and sustainable practices in herb sourcing is not just about the quality of the herbs but also about the broader impact on the environment and communities. By choosing sustainably harvested and ethically sourced herbs, you contribute to the preservation of plant species and the livelihoods of those who cultivate and harvest them. This approach aligns with a holistic view of health, emphasizing the interconnectedness of our well-being with the health of our planet.

When identifying high-quality herbs, there are several key indicators to look for. First, consider the visual appearance of the herbs. High-quality herbs should have vibrant colors and a healthy texture. For example, green herbs should be a rich, vibrant green rather than a dull, yellowish hue. The texture should be crisp, not wilted or brittle. These visual cues can give you a good indication of the herb's freshness.

Smell and taste are also important indicators of quality. Fresh herbs should have a strong, characteristic aroma. For instance, basil should smell sweet and peppery, while chamomile should have a gentle, apple-like scent. The taste should be potent and reflective of the herb's known flavor profile. An herb's lack of a strong smell or taste may be old or of poor quality.

Checking for signs of mold or pests is crucial. Mold can appear as white or greenish fuzz on the surface of the herbs, while pests may leave small holes or webs. Both can indicate poor storage conditions and compromise the herbs' safety and efficacy. Always scrutinize your herbs and avoid any that show signs of contamination.

Freshness is paramount for maintaining the potency of herbs. Fresh herbs retain their active compounds and provide the maximum therapeutic benefits. When purchasing fresh herbs, look for those harvested recently and stored correctly. For dried herbs, ensure they are stored in airtight containers away from light and moisture to preserve their potency.

Reputable sources for purchasing herbs are essential for ensuring quality. Specialty herbal stores and apothecaries often provide high-quality, carefully sourced herbs. These establishments usually have knowledgeable staff who can guide you in selecting the best herbs for your needs. Certified organic suppliers are another excellent option, as they adhere to strict standards for growing and processing herbs without synthetic pesticides or fertilizers.

Online retailers with good reputations can also be a reliable source of high-quality herbs. Look for retailers who provide detailed information about their sourcing and processing practices. Customer reviews and ratings can offer insights into the quality and reliability of the suppliers. Local farmers' markets and community-supported agriculture (CSA) programs are also fantastic places to find fresh, locally-grown herbs. These sources often emphasize sustainable and organic farming practices, ensuring that you get the best quality herbs while supporting local agriculture.

Certifications are crucial in ensuring the quality and ethical sourcing of herbs. USDA Organic certification indicates that the herbs are grown without synthetic pesticides, fertilizers, or genetically modified organisms (GMOs). This certification assures you that the herbs meet stringent organic standards. Fair Trade certification ensures that the farmers and workers involved in producing the herbs receive fair wages and work under safe conditions. This certification supports ethical labor practices and sustainable farming.

Good Manufacturing Practices (GMP) certification is another key indicator of quality. This certification ensures that the herbs are processed in facilities that adhere to high standards of cleanliness, consistency, and safety. GMP certification covers various aspects of production, including proper documentation, personnel training, and quality control procedures. Non-GMO Project verification indicates that the herbs are free from genetically modified organisms, aligning with a preference for natural, unaltered products.

By understanding these aspects of quality and sourcing, you can make informed choices when selecting herbs for your remedies. This knowledge empowers you to create potent, effective, and safe herbal preparations, ensuring that you and your loved ones can reap the full benefits of these ancient healing plants.

SAFETY PRECAUTIONS AND POTENTIAL SIDE EFFECTS

When it comes to herbal medicine, safety is paramount. It's easy to assume that because something is natural, it's inherently safe. However, this is not always the case. Natural does not equate to harmless. Many potent herbs can have side effects if not used correctly. Understanding proper dosage and methods of preparation is critical. For instance, too much of an herb like licorice root can lead to elevated blood pressure and potassium imbalances. Recognizing potential allergies and sensitivities is just as important. Some individuals may react to certain herbs with symptoms like rashes or itching. Always consult healthcare professionals before integrating new herbs, especially if you have pre-existing health conditions or are taking other medications.

Common side effects of herbs can vary widely. Gastrointestinal issues such as nausea and diarrhea are frequent complaints. For example, when taken internally, herbs like aloe vera can cause digestive upset if consumed in large quantities. Allergic reactions are another concern. Herbs like chamomile, which belongs to the ragweed family, can cause allergic responses in some people. These reactions might manifest as skin rashes, hives, or even more severe symptoms like difficulty breathing. Interactions with medications also pose significant risks. St. John's Wort, for instance, can reduce the efficacy of birth control pills and certain antidepressants. Signs of toxicity from overuse should not be ignored either. Herbs like comfrey, which contain pyrrolizidine alkaloids, can lead to liver damage if used excessively or improperly.

To use herbs safely, start with small doses and gradually increase as you monitor your body's response. This approach helps you gauge any potential adverse effects before they become severe. Keeping detailed records of your herbal use, including the types of herbs, dosages, and any reactions, can be invaluable. This practice helps identify patterns and provides useful information if you need to consult a healthcare professional. It's crucial to avoid using certain herbs during pregnancy and breastfeeding unless advised by a qualified practitioner. Herbs like pennyroyal and blue cohosh can induce labor or cause other complications. Staying informed about the latest research and safety guidelines ensures that you use herbs most effectively and safely.

Creating a safety checklist can be an excellent way to ensure you are using herbs responsibly. Start by verifying the identity of the herb. Misidentification can lead to the use of toxic plants by mistake. Always check for any contraindications with existing conditions or medications. For example, if you are on blood thinners, avoid herbs like ginkgo biloba, which can increase bleeding risk. Use proper preparation methods to maximize the efficacy and safety of the herb. Whether it's making tea, tincture, or salve, follow the recommended guidelines. Finally, monitor for any adverse effects. If you notice symptoms like nausea, dizziness, or skin reactions, discontinue use and consult a healthcare professional.

Safety Checklist

- Verify the identity of the herb
- Check for any contraindications with existing conditions or medications
- Use proper preparation methods
- Monitor for any adverse effects

This checklist can serve as a practical guide to help you safely navigate the complexities of herbal medicine. It's a valuable tool that encourages mindful and informed use of herbs, ensuring you reap their benefits without compromising your health.

ETHICAL HARVESTING AND SUSTAINABLE PRACTICES

When you gather herbs from the wild, it is vital to adhere to the principles of ethical harvesting. This approach protects plant populations and ensures that these resources remain available for future generations. Overharvesting is a major concern. Taking too much from one area can deplete local plant populations, making it difficult for them to regenerate. Instead, always harvest in a way that allows plants to continue growing and thriving. This means leaving enough behind for the plant to recover and produce seeds for the next season. By respecting wild habitats and ecosystems, you can help maintain the natural balance and biodiversity that these plants rely on.

Understanding the cultural significance of certain plants is also crucial. Many herbs have deep roots in indigenous traditions and are considered sacred. For instance, sage is not just a plant but a vital part of many Native American rituals. Harvesting such plants carelessly can be seen as disrespectful to the cultures that hold them dear. It's important to educate yourself about the cultural context of the herbs you use and ensure that your practices honor and respect these traditions.

Practical guidelines for ethical harvesting can help you gather herbs responsibly. Start by harvesting only what you need. This prevents waste and ensures that there is enough left for the plant to continue growing. Using proper tools, like sharp scissors or knives, minimizes damage to the plant and allows it to heal more quickly. Timing your harvest is another key factor. Harvest herbs at the right time of day and in the correct season for optimal potency and regrowth. For example, many herbs are best harvested in the morning after the dew has dried but before the day's heat sets in. Finally, always leave enough plants behind to ensure future growth. A good rule of thumb is to take no more than one-third of the plant or plant population in any given area.

Sustainable practices go beyond just how you harvest herbs; they also encompass how you support the broader ecosystem. Supporting local and sustainable farmers is one way to ensure that your herbs are grown in an environmentally friendly manner. These farmers often use organic methods and avoid harmful pesticides and chemicals. Choosing organically grown herbs benefits the environment and ensures that your herbal remedies are free from harmful residues. Participating in community-supported agriculture (CSA) programs is another way to support local, sustainable farming. These programs provide a direct connection between you and the farmers, ensuring transparency and quality in the herbs you receive. Promoting biodiversity in your herb garden also contributes to sustainability. By growing a variety of plants, you create a resilient ecosystem that supports beneficial insects and prevents soil depletion.

Ethical considerations in herbal use extend to the social and cultural dimensions. Understanding indigenous rights and traditional knowledge is paramount. Many traditional herbal practices are based on centuries-old wisdom passed down through generations. When you use these herbs, it's important to acknowledge and respect the source of this knowledge. Supporting fair trade and ethical sourcing practices ensures that the people who grow and harvest these herbs are treated fairly and compensated justly. This approach aligns with a holistic view of health, recognizing that the well-being of the people and communities involved in herbal production is as important as the quality of the herbs themselves.

Another important consideration is avoiding cultural appropriation in herbal practices. Cultural appropriation occurs when

CHAPTER 7: SAFETY AND SUSTAINABILITY IN HERBAL M...

elements of one culture are taken and used by another, often without permission or understanding. This can be particularly harmful when it comes to sacred or traditional practices. Educating yourself on the cultural significance of certain herbs and their traditional uses helps you avoid this pitfall. Seek out sources and practitioners from the cultures these herbs originate from and approach these practices with humility and respect.

By incorporating these principles into your herbal practices, you not only create effective and safe remedies but also contribute to the sustainability and ethical integrity of herbal medicine. This holistic approach ensures that your use of herbs is beneficial not only to you but also to the environment and the communities that cultivate these plants.

INTEGRATING MODERN SCIENCE WITH TRADITIONAL WISDOM

Combining traditional herbal wisdom with modern scientific research enriches the practice of herbal medicine. Traditional uses of herbs passed down through generations often lack the scientific validation that modern medicine demands. Integrating scientific research helps validate these traditional uses, making them more credible and widely accepted. For instance, traditional healers have long used turmeric for its anti-inflammatory properties. Modern science has confirmed these benefits, identifying curcumin as the active compound responsible for its therapeutic effects. This validation not only enhances the credibility of traditional practices but also encourages their integration into mainstream healthcare.

Scientific research also enhances the effectiveness of herbal remedies. By understanding the active compounds within herbs, scientists can optimize extraction methods to ensure maximum potency. For example, research on the best solvents for extracting certain compounds can lead to more effective tinctures and extracts. This scientific insight allows for the refinement of traditional remedies, making them more effective and reliable. Additionally, research helps identify synergistic effects between different herbs, enabling the creation of more potent herbal blends. This scientific approach bridges the gap between traditional and modern healthcare, providing a more holistic approach to treatment.

Ensuring the safety and efficacy of herbal remedies is another critical benefit of integrating modern science with traditional wisdom. Scientific studies can identify potential side effects and interactions with other medications, providing guidelines for safe use. For example, while St. John's Wort is effective for treating mild depression, research has shown it can interact negatively with certain medications, such as birth control pills and antidepressants. By understanding these interactions, healthcare providers can offer more informed advice, ensuring the safe use of herbal remedies. This approach helps mitigate risks and enhances the overall safety profile of herbal medicine.

Bridging the gap between traditional and modern healthcare involves more than just scientific validation. It requires a collaborative approach where traditional healers and modern healthcare professionals work together. Traditional healers bring invaluable experiential knowledge, while scientists contribute rigorous methodologies and analytical tools. This collaboration can lead to the development of new treatments that are both effective and culturally respectful. For instance, integrating acupuncture, a traditional Chinese practice, with conventional pain management techniques has led to more comprehensive pain relief strategies. This holistic approach benefits patients by offering a wider range of treatment options.

Key areas of scientific research that support traditional herbal practices include:

- Clinical studies on the efficacy of specific herbs.
- Research on the active compounds in herbs.
- Studies on the safety and potential side effects of herbs.

Clinical studies provide empirical evidence that supports the therapeutic claims of traditional herbs. For example, numerous clinical trials have confirmed the effectiveness of echinacea in reducing the duration and severity of colds. Research on active compounds helps identify the specific constituents responsible for an herb's medicinal properties. This knowledge allows for the standardization of herbal products, ensuring consistent quality and potency.

Studies on the safety and potential side effects of herbs are crucial for informing safe use. These studies help identify any adverse effects and provide guidelines for avoiding them. Advances in herbal extraction and preparation methods also significantly enhance the practice of herbal medicine. Techniques such as supercritical fluid extraction and ultrasonic-assisted extraction offer more efficient ways to obtain active compounds from herbs, resulting in more potent and effective products. These advancements make it possible to produce high-quality herbal remedies that meet modern standards of efficacy and safety.

Evidence-based approaches are essential in herbal medicine because they provide reliable and consistent results. This consistency builds trust and credibility in herbal practices, encouraging more people to adopt these natural treatments. Evidence-based approaches also inform safe and effective dosages, reducing the risk of adverse effects. By providing clear guidelines, evidence-based medicine helps integrate herbal treatments into mainstream healthcare. This integration is vital for offering patients a more comprehensive range of treatment options, blending the best of both traditional and modern practices.

Practical examples of how traditional wisdom and modern science can be combined include:

- Using scientific research to refine traditional remedies.
- Incorporating modern extraction techniques with traditional preparations.
- Consulting both traditional healers and modern healthcare professionals.

For instance, scientific research has refined the traditional use of ginseng by identifying optimal extraction methods and dosages. Modern extraction techniques, such as cold-pressing for essential oils, enhance the potency of traditional preparations. Consulting both traditional healers and modern healthcare professionals ensures a holistic approach to treatment, combining experiential knowledge with scientific rigor. Staying updated with the latest research and developments is also crucial for maintaining the relevance and efficacy of herbal medicine. This ongoing education helps practitioners adapt to new findings and continually improve their practices.

CREATING A SUSTAINABLE HERBAL GARDEN

Growing your herbs at home offers numerous benefits, both for the environment and your personal health. One of the most significant advantages is reducing the carbon footprint associated with herb sourcing. When you grow your herbs, you eliminate the need for transportation and packaging, which contribute to greenhouse gas emissions. This small step can make a big difference in the fight against climate change. Additionally, having a sustainable herbal garden ensures you have a fresh and consistent supply of herbs. There's nothing like stepping outside and picking fresh basil or mint for your tea or recipe. The freshness of home-grown herbs also means they retain more of their beneficial properties, offering you the best possible health benefits.

Promoting biodiversity and ecosystem health is another compelling reason to start your herbal garden. By growing a variety of plants, you create a mini-ecosystem that supports beneficial insects like bees and butterflies. These pollinators are essential for the health of our natural environment. Moreover, a diverse garden helps maintain soil health by preventing nutrient depletion. Growing your herbs also enhances your personal connection with nature and herbal practices. Tending to a garden can be a meditative and rewarding experience, allowing you to engage with the natural world meaningfully. This hands-on approach deepens your understanding of the plants you use for healing, making your herbal practice more holistic and fulfilling.

Starting a sustainable herbal garden involves several practical steps. First, choose the right location and soil for herb growth. Most herbs prefer well-drained soil and plenty of sunlight, so select a spot in your garden that gets at least six to eight hours of direct sunlight daily. If your soil is heavy or clay-like, consider amending it with compost or sand to improve drainage. Raised beds can also be an excellent option for controlling soil quality and drainage. Next, select herbs that are well-suited to your local climate. For example, Mediterranean herbs like rosemary and thyme thrive in hot, dry conditions, while herbs like mint and parsley prefer cooler, moist environments. Researching the specific needs of each herb will help you create a thriving garden.

Using organic and sustainable gardening practices is crucial for maintaining a healthy garden and protecting the environment.

Avoid synthetic pesticides and fertilizers, which can harm beneficial insects and contaminate soil and water. Instead, opt for organic compost and natural pest control methods. Implementing water conservation techniques is also essential. Drip irrigation systems or soaker hoses deliver water directly to the plant roots, reducing evaporation and ensuring efficient water use. Mulching around your plants helps retain soil moisture and reduce weed growth.

Certain herbs are particularly well-suited for home gardens due to their versatility and ease of growth. Basil is a fantastic choice for both culinary and medicinal uses. It's great in salads, pesto, and teas and offers anti-inflammatory and antibacterial properties. Mint is another excellent herb to grow at home. It's perfect for digestive health, making it a staple for teas and infusions. However, mint can be invasive, so it's best grown in pots or containers. Calendula is a beautiful and useful herb known for its skin-healing properties. Its bright orange flowers can be used in salves, creams, and teas. Echinacea, famed for its immune-supporting properties, is another valuable addition to your garden. It produces stunning purple flowers and can be used to make teas and tinctures.

Maintaining garden sustainability involves several ongoing practices. Composting and soil enrichment are fundamental. Adding compost to your soil improves its structure, fertility, and water-holding capacity. You can create your compost from kitchen scraps, yard waste, and other organic materials. Natural pest control methods, such as introducing beneficial insects like ladybugs and using neem oil, can help keep harmful pests at bay without using chemicals. Crop rotation and companion planting are also essential techniques. Rotating crops yearly prevents soil depletion and reduces the risk of disease. Companion planting involves growing certain plants together that benefit each other.

CHAPTER 7: SAFETY AND SUSTAINABILITY IN HERBAL M... 123

For example, planting basil near tomatoes can help repel pests and improve growth.

Harvesting practices that promote regrowth are vital for a sustainable garden. Always use clean, sharp tools to harvest your herbs, making clean cuts that minimize damage to the plant. Harvest in the morning after the dew has dried for the best flavor and potency. Avoid taking more than one-third of the plant at any time to ensure it can continue growing and producing. This approach ensures that your garden remains productive and healthy year after year, providing you with a steady supply of fresh, potent herbs.

NAVIGATING HERBAL INTERACTIONS WITH CONVENTIONAL MEDICATIONS

Understanding herb-drug interactions is crucial for anyone integrating herbal remedies with conventional medications. This knowledge helps prevent adverse reactions, ensuring both the herbs and medications work effectively. For example, taking St. John's Wort while on antidepressants can reduce the medication's effectiveness, potentially leading to a relapse of depressive symptoms. Being aware of such interactions safeguards your overall health and well-being. Additionally, understanding these interactions enhances communication with healthcare providers. When you discuss your herbal and conventional treatments openly with your doctor, they can guide you in making safe and effective choices.

Common herb-drug interactions can pose significant risks if not properly managed. St. John's Wort, a popular herb for treating mild depression, can interact with antidepressants, reducing their efficacy and potentially leading to withdrawal symptoms. Ginkgo Biloba, often used to improve cognitive function, can increase the risk of bleeding when taken with blood thinners like warfarin. Licorice root, known for its soothing properties, can raise blood pressure when combined with certain blood pressure medications. Echinacea is often used to boost the immune system but can interfere with immunosuppressants, potentially compromising their effectiveness. These examples highlight the importance of being vigilant about the herbs you use, especially if you are on conventional medications.

To safely combine herbs with conventional medications, start by consulting healthcare professionals before introducing any new herb into your regimen. They can provide personalized advice based on your specific health conditions and medications. Keeping detailed records of all herbs and medications you are using is another essential practice. This record can help you and your healthcare provider identify potential interactions and adjust your treatments accordingly. Monitoring for any signs of adverse reactions, such as unusual symptoms or changes in your health, is crucial. If you notice anything amiss, consult your healthcare provider immediately. Adjusting dosages as needed under professional guidance ensures that both your herbal and conventional treatments are effective and safe.

Creating a reference chart for common interactions can be a valuable tool for managing your herbal and medication use. This chart should list herbs and their known interactions with specific medications, providing brief descriptions of potential side effects. For instance, you could include that St. John's Wort may reduce the effectiveness of birth control pills and antidepressants or that Ginkgo Biloba can increase bleeding risk when taken with blood thinners. Offering general recommendations for safe use, such as avoiding certain herbs if you are on specific medications, can guide your decisions. Encouraging regular consultation with healthcare providers ensures that you stay informed and make safe choices.

Herb-Drug Interaction Chart

- **Herb:** St. John's Wort
  - **Interacts with:** Antidepressants, birth control pills
  - **Potential side effects:** Reduced medication efficacy, withdrawal symptoms
  - **Recommendation:** Consult healthcare provider before use
- **Herb:** Ginkgo Biloba
  - **Interacts with** Blood thinners (e.g., warfarin)
  - **Potential side effects:** Increased risk of bleeding
  - **Recommendation:** Monitor closely, consult a healthcare provider
- **Herb:** Licorice Root
  - **Interacts with** Blood pressure medications
  - **Potential side effects:** Elevated blood pressure
  - **Recommendation:** Use with caution, consult a healthcare provider
- **Herb:** Echinacea
  - **Interacts with** Immunosuppressants
  - **Potential side effects:** Reduced medication efficacy
  - **Recommendation:** Avoid if on immunosuppressants; consult a healthcare provider

This simple chart can serve as a quick reference, helping you navigate the complexities of herb-drug interactions. Keeping it handy allows you to make informed decisions and ensures that your herbal and conventional treatments work harmoniously.

Incorporating this knowledge into your daily practice not only enhances the safety and effectiveness of your treatments but also empowers you to take an active role in managing your health. By understanding potential interactions and consulting with healthcare providers, you can confidently integrate herbal remedies into your wellness routine, enjoying the best of both traditional and modern medicine.

As we move forward, the next chapter will delve into building a holistic lifestyle, where we explore daily rituals, dietary changes, and the mind-body connection to further enhance your well-being.

CHAPTER 8: BUILDING A HOLISTIC LIFESTYLE

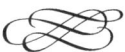

The first time I truly understood the power of daily rituals, I was living in a small mountain village, far removed from the hustle and bustle of city life. Each morning, the villagers would gather by a bubbling stream to start their day with a simple yet profound ritual: sipping a warm herbal tea while listening to the gentle sounds of nature. This daily practice created a sense of peace and connection, setting a calm tone for the day ahead. It was then that I realized the transformative power of incorporating small, consistent practices into our lives.

DAILY RITUALS FOR HOLISTIC HEALTH

Daily rituals can significantly enhance your overall health and well-being by creating a sense of structure and stability in your life. These practices help anchor your day, providing a sense of predictability and security amidst the chaos of modern living. By establishing regular routines, you can promote mindfulness and intentional living, allowing you to approach each day with a clear sense of purpose and focus. These rituals also enhance your physical, emotional, and spiritual health by integrating small, consistent practices that yield long-term benefits.

One of the simplest yet most effective daily rituals involving herbs is starting your day with a cleansing herbal tea. This practice not only hydrates your body but also infuses it with the healing properties of various herbs. For instance, a morning tea made with lemon and ginger can aid in detoxification, stimulate digestion, and boost your immune system. As you sip your tea, take a moment to set your intentions for the day, grounding yourself in the present moment.

In the evening, incorporating an herbal bath can help you unwind and prepare for a restful night's sleep. A bath infused with lavender and chamomile can soothe your muscles, calm your mind, and promote deep relaxation. The warm water opens your pores, allowing the beneficial compounds from the herbs to penetrate deeply into your skin. This practice not only provides physical relief but also serves as a mental and emotional reset, washing away the stresses of the day.

Another powerful ritual is using herbal oils for morning self-massage, known as Abhyanga in Ayurvedic tradition. This practice involves massaging warm oil infused with herbs like sesame or coconut oil into your skin. It enhances circulation, nourishes your skin, and promotes a sense of calm and balance. The act of self-massage also fosters a deep connection with your body, allowing you to start your day with a sense of self-love and care.

Creating a bedtime routine with calming herbal infusions can significantly improve your sleep quality. A cup of chamomile or valerian tea before bed can help you relax and drift off to sleep more easily. Pair this with a few minutes of deep breathing or meditation to quiet your mind and prepare your body for rest.

This nightly ritual can become a cherished part of your day, signaling to your body that it's time to unwind and recharge.

To establish these daily rituals, it's important to set aside dedicated time each day. Choose moments that fit seamlessly into your routine, whether it's the quiet of the early morning or the calm of the evening. Personalize these rituals to suit your needs and preferences, making them enjoyable and sustainable. Use reminders and cues, such as a favorite mug for your morning tea or a special candle for your evening bath, to stay consistent. Journaling the effects and benefits of these rituals can also be incredibly helpful. Reflect on how these practices make you feel, noting any changes in your physical, emotional, and spiritual well-being.

For instance, you might start your day with a lemon and ginger tea for detoxification, followed by a midday mindfulness break with peppermint tea to refresh your mind. In the evening, indulge in a lavender bath to relax your muscles and calm your spirit. Finally, end your day with a cup of chamomile tea and a few minutes of meditation to prepare for a restful night's sleep.

By incorporating these daily rituals into your life, you can create a foundation of health and well-being that supports you through the challenges and joys of each day. These small, consistent practices not only enhance your physical health but also nurture your emotional and spiritual well-being, helping you lead a balanced and fulfilling life.

COMBINING HERBAL REMEDIES WITH MEDITATION AND YOGA

There is a unique synergy that unfolds when you combine herbal remedies with meditation and yoga. These practices, when integrated, amplify each other's benefits, resulting in a more profound sense of well-being. Imagine starting your day with a calming cup of Tulsi tea, which is known for its ability to enhance mental clarity and focus. As you sip, you feel a sense of calm enveloping you, preparing your mind for a focused and peaceful meditation session. This practice not only enhances relaxation and stress relief but also supports a balanced state of physical and mental health. The herbs act as natural allies, deepening your mindfulness and spiritual connection, thereby promoting holistic health and well-being.

Tulsi, also known as Holy Basil, is one of the key herbs that perfectly complements meditation and yoga. It is revered for its ability to clear the mind and enhance focus, making it an ideal companion for your meditative practices. Ashwagandha, another powerful herb, is known for its grounding properties and ability to reduce stress. Incorporating Ashwagandha into your routine can help you feel more centered and balanced, making it easier to achieve a state of calm during meditation. Peppermint is excellent for enhancing breath awareness, a crucial aspect of both yoga and meditation. Its invigorating scent can help you stay present and mindful of each breath. Lavender, with its soothing aroma, promotes relaxation and can be particularly beneficial during evening practices.

To seamlessly integrate these herbs into your meditation and yoga routines, consider drinking herbal tea before you begin. A cup of Tulsi tea can clear your mind and prepare you for a focused meditation session. During yoga, using essential oils can enhance relaxation and deepen your practice. A few drops of lavender oil on your yoga mat or diffused in the room can create a calming atmosphere, helping you to relax more deeply into each pose. Herbal incense is another effective way to incorporate herbs into your meditation space. Burning incense made from calming herbs like sandalwood or lavender can create a serene environment conducive to deep meditation. After your yoga practice, an herbal bath can provide a perfect end to your routine, aiding in muscle recovery and enhancing relaxation. A bath infused with chamomile and eucalyptus can soothe sore muscles and refresh your body.

For a morning yoga session, consider starting with a cup of peppermint tea. Its invigorating properties can awaken your senses and provide a gentle boost of energy, perfect for a revitalizing yoga practice. In the evening, a cup of Tulsi tea can help calm your mind, preparing you for a peaceful meditation session. Using lavender essential oil during your yoga practice can promote relaxation, helping you to unwind and release tension. After meditation, treat yourself to an herbal bath with chamomile and eucalyptus. The combination of these herbs can relax your muscles, clear your mind, and prepare you for a restful night's sleep.

Combining herbal remedies with meditation and yoga creates a holistic practice that nurtures your body, mind, and spirit. The herbs enhance the benefits of these ancient practices, deepening your sense of relaxation, balance, and overall well-being. Through these integrated rituals, you can cultivate a lifestyle that supports your health and enriches your daily experience.

DIETARY CHANGES TO COMPLEMENT HERBAL TREATMENTS

Understanding the impact of diet on holistic health is crucial. Your dietary choices play a significant role in supporting the body's natural healing processes. When you consume whole, nutrient-dense foods, you provide your body with the essential building blocks it needs to function optimally. This, in turn, enhances the absorption and efficacy of the herbs you incorporate into your regimen. A balanced diet complements herbal treatments by promoting overall nutritional balance and wellness. Aligning your diet with specific health goals and herbal remedies can amplify the benefits you receive from both.

To create a diet that complements herbal treatments, emphasize whole, unprocessed foods. These foods are rich in essential nutrients and free from harmful additives. Include a variety of fruits, vegetables, and whole grains to ensure you get a broad spectrum of vitamins, minerals, and antioxidants. Minimizing sugar, caffeine, and processed foods is also crucial, as these can interfere with your body's ability to absorb nutrients and disrupt your natural energy balance. Staying hydrated is essential for overall health. Drink plenty of water and herbal teas throughout the day to keep your body well-hydrated and support the detoxification process.

Making dietary changes can be challenging, but with practical strategies, you can gradually transition to a healthier diet. Start by incorporating more whole foods into your meals. Replace refined grains with whole grains, and add an extra serving of vegetables to your plate. Planning balanced meals and snacks ahead of time can help you stay on track. Use herbs and spices to enhance the flavor and nutritional value of your dishes. For example, adding turmeric and ginger to your meals can provide anti-inflammatory benefits.

Keeping a food journal can be a helpful tool for tracking your progress and noting the benefits you experience from your dietary changes.

Consider specific dietary recommendations that align with your herbal treatments. An anti-inflammatory diet can be particularly beneficial if you're dealing with chronic pain or inflammatory conditions. Incorporate turmeric and ginger into your meals regularly. These potent herbs can help reduce inflammation and support joint health. Detoxifying meals can support your body's natural elimination processes. Dandelion greens and lemon are excellent choices for this purpose. Dandelion greens are rich in vitamins and minerals, while lemon aids digestion and detoxification. For immune-boosting benefits, include garlic, onions, and elderberries in your diet. Garlic and onions are known for their antimicrobial properties, and elderberries are rich in antioxidants that support immune function.

Calming foods can help manage stress and promote relaxation. Chamomile and oats are excellent choices for this purpose. Chamomile has soothing properties that can help calm the nervous system, while oats provide a steady source of energy and support serotonin production, which is essential for mood regulation. Incorporate these foods into your daily meals to experience their calming effects.

For breakfast, you might enjoy a bowl of oatmeal topped with fresh berries and a sprinkle of cinnamon. This meal provides a balanced start to your day, rich in fiber, antioxidants, and calming properties. At lunch, a salad made with dandelion greens, avocado, and a lemon vinaigrette can support detoxification and provide essential nutrients. Dinner could include a hearty vegetable stir-fry with garlic, onions, and turmeric-seasoned quinoa. This meal supports immune function and reduces inflammation. For a calming evening snack, enjoy a cup of chamomile tea with a small bowl of oatmeal cookies.

Integrating these dietary changes into your life can significantly enhance the effectiveness of your herbal treatments. By providing your body with the nutrients it needs to function optimally, you can support your natural healing processes and promote overall health and well-being. These changes don't have to be drastic; even small, consistent adjustments can lead to significant improvements over time.

MIND-BODY CONNECTION AND HERBAL MEDICINE

The connection between the mind and body is profound, influencing every aspect of your health. Mental and emotional states significantly affect physical health. Stress, anxiety, and depression can manifest as physical symptoms like headaches, muscle tension, and digestive issues. Conversely, physical health impacts mental and emotional well-being. Chronic pain or illness can lead to feelings of frustration, sadness, or anxiety. Stress plays a crucial role in chronic illness and overall health. It can exacerbate existing conditions, weaken the immune system, and disrupt sleep patterns. Adopting holistic approaches that address both mind and body can provide comprehensive benefits, improving your overall health and quality of life.

Herbs can play a vital role in supporting the mind-body connection. Ashwagandha is well-known for its ability to reduce stress and enhance physical vitality. It helps to balance cortisol levels, providing a calming effect while boosting energy. Rhodiola is another powerful herb that supports mental clarity and physical endurance. It is particularly effective in combating fatigue and enhancing cognitive function. Lavender is celebrated for its ability to promote emotional balance and relaxation. Its soothing properties can help alleviate anxiety and improve sleep quality. Peppermint is excellent for enhancing mental focus and also supports digestive health, making it a versatile addition to your herbal toolkit.

To enhance the mind-body connection, consider incorporating mindfulness and meditation into your daily routines. These practices help you stay present and aware, reducing stress and promoting a sense of calm. Using herbs to support mental clarity and emotional balance can further enhance these benefits. For example, drinking Ashwagandha tea before meditation can help ground you, making it easier to achieve a state of calm. Practicing yoga or tai chi can integrate physical and mental well-being, promoting flexibility, strength, and mental focus. Keeping a journal to reflect on your mind-body experiences can be incredibly insightful. Note how different practices and herbs affect your physical and emotional states, helping you tailor your routine for maximum benefit.

Specific examples of mind-body practices can make it easier to integrate these concepts into your life. Drinking Ashwagandha tea before meditation can help you feel grounded and centered, enhancing your focus and calm. Before a yoga session, taking a Rhodiola tincture can boost your endurance, allowing you to get the most out of your practice. Using lavender essential oil in a diffuser during relaxation exercises can create a calming atmosphere, helping you to release tension and relax deeply. For a midday refresh, a cup of peppermint tea can sharpen your mental focus while also aiding digestion, providing a holistic boost to your well-being.

By understanding and nurturing the mind-body connection, you can create a holistic approach to health that supports both your physical and emotional well-being. Integrating herbs into your daily practices can enhance these benefits, providing natural support for your overall health. Whether you are meditating, practicing yoga, or simply reflecting on your day, these practices and herbs can help you achieve a balanced and fulfilling life.

BUILDING A COMMUNITY AROUND HERBAL PRACTICES

Connecting with others who share an interest in herbal medicine can significantly enhance your practice and overall well-being. When you engage with a community, you open yourself up to a wealth of shared knowledge and experiences. This collective wisdom can provide new insights and techniques that you might not discover on your own. By sharing your own experiences and learning from others, you can deepen your understanding and refine your skills. The support and encouragement from a community can be incredibly motivating, especially when you encounter challenges or setbacks. Knowing that others have faced similar obstacles and found solutions can inspire you to keep going.

Building a sense of belonging and purpose is another profound benefit of community engagement. You feel connected and supported when you are part of a group with shared interests. This sense of belonging can enhance your overall well-being, providing emotional and mental benefits that complement the physical benefits of herbal medicine. Engaging with a community also offers opportunities for skill development. Whether you are attending workshops, participating in study groups, or collaborating on projects, you continuously learn and grow. This ongoing education can keep your practice fresh and exciting, preventing stagnation and fostering a lifelong passion for herbal medicine.

There are many ways to connect with others who are interested in herbal medicine. Joining local herbalist groups or clubs is a great starting point. These groups often have regular meetings, workshops, and events where you can learn and share with like-minded individuals. Participating in online forums and social media groups can also be valuable, especially if you live in an area with limited local resources. These platforms provide a space to ask questions, share experiences, and access a global community of herbal enthusiasts. Attending workshops, classes, and conferences can offer in-depth learning opportunities and the chance to meet experts in the field. Hosting or joining herbal study groups and meetups allows for more intimate, hands-on learning experiences.

To actively participate and contribute to the herbal community, start by sharing your personal experiences and successes. Your journey can inspire others and provide practical insights. Don't hesitate to ask questions and seek advice; this openness fosters a collaborative and supportive environment. Volunteering for community herbal projects, such as helping to maintain a community herb garden or participating in local health fairs, can also be rewarding. Collaborating on herbal research and projects, whether through formal studies or informal group experiments, can deepen your knowledge and contribute to the broader field of herbal medicine.

Consider organizing activities that build a community around herbal practices. An herbal foraging walk can be a wonderful way to connect with nature and learn about local plants. Invite a knowledgeable guide to lead the walk and share insights about the herbs you encounter. Hosting a herbal tea-tasting event can be a delightful way to explore the different flavors and benefits of various teas. Encourage participants to bring their favorite blends and share recipes. Participating in a community garden project allows you to work alongside others, growing and tending to medicinal herbs. This hands-on experience can enhance your understanding of plant cultivation and provide a sense of accomplishment. Leading a workshop on making herbal remedies, such as tinctures, salves, or infusions, can be a fulfilling way to share your knowledge and skills. Provide step-by-step instructions and encourage participants to ask questions and share their experiences.

Building a community around herbal practices not only enriches your own experience but also contributes to the collective knowledge and well-being of the group. By engaging with others, you create a supportive network that fosters growth, learning, and a deeper connection to the healing power of plants.

CONTINUING YOUR JOURNEY: FURTHER RESOURCES AND READING

Ongoing learning in herbal medicine is crucial for deepening your knowledge and honing your skills. The field of herbal medicine is dynamic, with new research and developments emerging regularly. Staying updated with the latest studies can enhance your understanding of how herbs work and their potential benefits. This continuous education not only builds your confidence but also equips you with the expertise to explore new herbs and practices. Whether you are a beginner or a seasoned practitioner, there is always something new to learn.

To support your journey, several key resources can provide invaluable information and insights. Comprehensive herb guides and textbooks offer detailed descriptions of various herbs, their properties, and uses. Books like "The Herbal Medicine-Maker's Handbook" by James Green and "The Complete Herbal Tutor" by Anne McIntyre are excellent starting points. Online courses and webinars from reputable institutions, such as the American Herbalists

Guild, provide structured learning opportunities and access to expert knowledge. Websites and blogs run by experienced herbalists can also be rich sources of practical advice and tips. Additionally, peer-reviewed journals and scientific publications, such as the "Journal of Herbal Medicine," offer evidence-based information that can enhance your practice.

When it comes to effective learning, setting clear goals and objectives is essential. Determine what you want to achieve with your herbal studies, whether it's mastering the use of specific herbs, understanding herbal formulations, or learning about the historical context of herbal medicine. Creating a study schedule and staying consistent can help you manage your time effectively and make steady progress. Joining study groups or forums can provide a supportive environment for discussion and exchange of ideas. Applying new knowledge through practice and experimentation is also crucial. Try making your own tinctures, teas, or salves and observe their effects. This hands-on experience will deepen your understanding and build your confidence.

To help you get started, here is a curated list of recommended resources. "The Herbal Medicine-Maker's Handbook" by James Green is a practical guide that covers everything from basic preparations to advanced techniques. "The Complete Herbal Tutor" by Anne McIntyre provides a comprehensive overview of herbal medicine, including detailed profiles of numerous herbs. The American Herbalists Guild offers an excellent online course that covers various aspects of herbal practice. The website Learning-Herbs.com is a great resource for beginners and experienced practitioners alike, offering tutorials, articles, and community support. For those interested in scientific research, the "Journal of Herbal Medicine" publishes peer-reviewed studies on the efficacy and safety of herbal treatments.

By continuously educating yourself and exploring new resources, you can deepen your understanding of herbal medicine and enhance your practice. This ongoing learning not only builds your confidence and expertise but also allows you to stay abreast of new developments and innovations in the field. Whether you are reading a new book, taking an online course, or experimenting with new herbs, each step you take brings you closer to mastering the art of herbal medicine.

As you continue to expand your knowledge and skills, remember that the journey of learning is ongoing. There is always more to discover, new herbs to explore, and new techniques to master. Embrace this continuous journey with curiosity and enthusiasm, knowing that each step you take brings you closer to a deeper understanding of the healing power of herbs. By investing in your education and staying open to new experiences, you can create a fulfilling and enriching practice that supports your health and well-being.

CONCLUSION

Throughout this journey, we've explored the profound wisdom embedded in the traditions of Native American and Traditional Chinese Medicine. These ancient practices, steeped in rich cultural contexts, have significantly contributed to the field of herbal medicine. Whether it's the spiritual connection Native Americans have with their sacred herbs or the philosophical underpinnings of Traditional Chinese Medicine, both traditions offer invaluable insights into holistic healing.

By comparing these two practices, we've seen how Native American medicine emphasizes spiritual rituals and the use of local plants like sage and sweetgrass, while Traditional Chinese Medicine (TCM) focuses on balancing yin and yang and harnessing the power of qi through herbs like ginseng and astragalus. Despite their differences, both traditions share a common goal: achieving harmony within the body and between the individual and their environment.

In this book, we've delved into detailed profiles of key herbs from Native American, Traditional Chinese, and other ancient cultures around the world. From the immune-boosting properties of echinacea to the vitality-enhancing effects of ginseng, each herb has been carefully examined for its historical significance and modern applications. We've also provided practical recipes and methods for making herbal teas, tinctures, salves, ointments, syrups, essential oils, and other preparations. These time-tested remedies can be seamlessly integrated into your daily routine, offering natural solutions to common health challenges.

Modern scientific research has played a crucial role in validating the effectiveness and safety of these ancient remedies. By bridging traditional wisdom with contemporary science, we've ensured that the practices and recipes shared in this book are both credible and reliable. This integration reinforces the therapeutic benefits of herbal medicine, making it a trustworthy addition to your health regimen.

Ethical sourcing and sustainable practices are paramount when it comes to herbal medicine. We've outlined guidelines for identifying high-quality herbs, sourcing them responsibly, and using them safely. By adhering to these principles, you not only ensure the potency and safety of your remedies but also contribute to the preservation of our natural resources and respect for cultural traditions.

Incorporating herbal remedies into a holistic lifestyle requires a multifaceted approach. We've discussed how daily rituals, dietary changes, and mind-body practices can enhance the efficacy of herbs and promote overall well-being. Simple practices like starting your day with a cleansing herbal tea or winding down with a relaxing lavender bath can make a significant difference in your health.

Building a community around herbal practices is equally important. Sharing knowledge, experiences, and support with like-minded individuals can enrich your journey and foster a deeper understanding of herbal medicine. Whether through local herbalist groups, online forums, or community workshops, engaging with others can provide valuable insights and encouragement.

This book equips you with comprehensive knowledge and practical skills to use ancient remedies effectively and safely. By embracing these practices, you empower yourself to take control of your health and achieve self-sufficiency. Respecting cultural traditions and practicing sustainability is integral to this journey, ensuring that this ancient wisdom is preserved for future generations.

The information presented in this book is backed by thorough research and credible sources, giving you the confidence to integrate these remedies into your life. I encourage you to experiment with the recipes and methods provided, customizing them to suit your needs and preferences. Join or build a community around herbal practices to share knowledge, support each other, and continue learning.

Pursuing further education in herbal medicine can deepen your understanding and enhance your skills. The resources and ongoing research recommended in this book are excellent starting points for your continued learning.

Embracing natural health solutions can be a transformative experience. By reviving ancient remedies, you not only enhance your well-being but also preserve valuable cultural knowledge. Embark on a journey of self-discovery and holistic healing, using the wisdom of ancient herbal traditions as your guide.

Thank you for joining me on this journey through the world of ancient remedies. Stay curious, open-minded, and committed to your health and well-being. I am confident that you will find lasting benefits in the knowledge and practices shared in this book. Here's to a healthier, more balanced life through the power of natural healing.

Your review matters! Please take time to review this guide. Your message and experience using Ancient Remedies Revived can help others struggling with health concerns or fears. By sharing your practical and effective solutions, you can inspire and empower others to take charge of their health and embrace natural remedies.

REFERENCES

Indigenous Native American Healing Traditions - PMC https://www.ncbi.nlm.nih.gov/pmc/articles/PMC2913884/

Philosophical Basis of Traditional Chinese Medicine http://www.china.org.cn/english/MATERIAL/185381.htm

A Comparison of Chinese and American Indian (Chumash) ... https://www.ncbi.nlm.nih.gov/pmc/articles/PMC2862936/

Trading Medicinal Plants in the Ancient World https://unitedplantsavers.org/trading-medicinal-plants-in-the-ancient-world/

The Four Sacred Herbs | Duke Gardens https://gardens.duke.edu/four-sacred-herbs

Traditional Medicine: Cedar https://www.creehealth.org/health-tips/traditional-medicine-cedar

Tea Recipes From The Sioux Chef's Indigenous Kitchen https://www.cowboysindians.com/2017/10/tea-recipes-from-the-sioux-chefs-indigenous-kitchen/

How to Make Homemade Calendula Salve for Healthy Skin https://homesteadandchill.com/homemade-calendula-salve-recipe/

Traditional Chinese Medicine Herbs List to Improve Overall ... https://wthn.com/blogs/wthnside-out/traditional-chinese-medicine-herbs-list?srsltid=AfmBOopyBQ-oVOLZpxAx3eFDDK1TaphvlbazT3NeA9u01xO1Au02SF9G

Adaptogenic effects of Panax ginseng on modulation ... https://www.ncbi.nlm.nih.gov/pmc/articles/PMC7322748/

Preparing Herbal Decoctions https://www.cmro.gov.hk/html/eng/useful_information/public_health/pamphlet/Preparing_Herbal_Decoctions.html

Traditional Chinese Medicine to Boost your Immune System https://herbal-inn.com/blogs/blog/traditional-chinese-medicine-boost-immune-system

Ayurvedic herbs: Benefits, uses, evidence, precautions https://www.medicalnewstoday.com/articles/ayurvedic-herbs

Traditional ancient Egyptian medicine: A review - PMC https://www.ncbi.nlm.nih.gov/pmc/articles/PMC8459052/

Indigenous Uses, Phytochemical Analysis, and Anti- ... https://www.ncbi.nlm.nih.gov/pmc/articles/PMC9231311/

Traditional Medicines in Africa: An Appraisal of Ten Potent ... https://www.ncbi.nlm.nih.gov/pmc/articles/PMC3866779/

The Art of the Herbal Bath https://aromaticmedicineschool.com/the-art-of-the-herbal-bath

REFERENCES

Herbal Cough Syrup Recipe for a Dry Cough https://theherbalacademy.com/blog/herbal-cough-syrup-recipe-for-a-dry-cough/

A Comprehensive Guide to Essential Oil Extraction Methods https://www.newdirectionsaromatics.com/blog/articles/how-essential-oils-are-made.html

How to Make Lotion with Herbal Ingredients https://www.learningherbs.com/blog/how-to-make-lotion

The growing use of herbal medicines: issues relating to ... https://www.ncbi.nlm.nih.gov/pmc/articles/PMC3887317/

Astragalus Root and Elderberry Fruit Extracts Enhance the ... https://www.ncbi.nlm.nih.gov/pmc/articles/PMC3484152/

Decoction - an overview https://www.sciencedirect.com/topics/agricultural-and-biological-sciences/decoction

30 Herbs That Fight Cold And Flu https://www.prevention.com/health/g20493406/30-herbs-that-fight-cold-and-flu/

Advancing herbal medicine: enhancing product quality and ... https://www.ncbi.nlm.nih.gov/pmc/articles/PMC10561302/

Herbs & Spices Program: Joint Rainforest Alliance and ... https://www.rainforest-alliance.org/business/certification/herbs-and-spices-program/

The growing use of herbal medicines: issues relating to ... https://www.ncbi.nlm.nih.gov/pmc/articles/PMC3887317/

Herb-Drug Interactions | NCCIH https://www.nccih.nih.gov/health/providers/digest/herb-drug-interactions

A Comparison of Chinese and American Indian (Chumash) ... https://www.ncbi.nlm.nih.gov/pmc/articles/PMC2862936/

Traditional medicine has a long history of contributing to ... https://www.who.int/news-room/feature-stories/detail/traditional-medicine-has-a-long-history-of-contributing-to-conventional-medicine-and-continues-to-hold-promise

6 Ways to Incorporate Medicinal Herbs Into Your Daily ... https://richmondnaturalmed.com/medicinal-herbs-daily-routine/

Find Inner Peace with these Five Herbs for Meditation https://www.gaiaherbs.com/blogs/seeds-of-knowledge/find-inner-peace-with-these-five-herbs-for-meditation?srsltid=AfmBOopnpsO56RtGsaoZoJ0dIDmuo_3mH83c774n5SnRwSsMsEbkvBr6

Made in the USA
Coppell, TX
15 December 2024

42698643R10085